THE THEORETICAL BASIS
OF
NURSING

The *slinky*® was used as the basis for the illustrations in this
book through the courtesy of James Industries, Inc.

An Introduction to

THE THEORETICAL BASIS
OF
NURSING

Martha E. Rogers, B.S., A.M., M.P.H., Sc.D., R.N.

Head, Division of Nurse Education
School of Education
New York University
New York

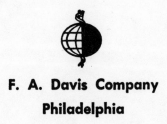

F. A. Davis Company
Philadelphia

Library of Congress Catalog Card Number 71-105539
ISBN 0-8036-7490-2

FOREWORD

People are at the center of nursing's purpose. The science of nursing is directed toward describing the life process in man and toward explaining and predicting the nature and direction of its development. Nursing's hypothetical generalizations and unifying principles emerge out of abstract thought within the framework of nursing's conceptual system and find verification in scientific research and logical analysis. A conceptual model of man provides a way of perceiving the life process and establishes a foundation for continuing development of relevant research and significant utilization of investigatory findings.

Nursing is a humanistic science dedicated to compassionate concern for maintaining and promoting health, preventing illness, and caring for and rehabilitating the sick and disabled. Man, whom nursing strives to serve, is a unified whole, a synergistic system, who cannot be explained by knowledge of his parts. Sweeping changes taking place throughout the world emphasize life's creativity and challenge the most visionary to foretell the days ahead. The goals of achieving human health and welfare have taken on undreamed-of dimensions as man's earth-bound past merges with his space-directed future.

The preparation of this volume has been motivated by a deep-seated conviction of the critical need for nursing practice to be underwritten by substantive knowledge so that human beings may benefit. Its contents are organized into three units. Unit I is the story of man's evolution through time, thus providing a backdrop for examining contemporary thoughts and theories about man. Unit II presents the basic assumptions which are proposed to underlie nursing's conceptual system. In Unit III a design is developed for nursing's abstract system. Guiding principles, postulated to depict the nature of life's becoming, are enunciated. Verifying evidence of conceptual validity is presented, and potentially fruitful and much-needed areas of further research are suggested. The social significance of nursing comes into view as nursing's body of scientific knowledge is translated into practice.

Escalating scientific and technological advances are forcing new explanations of man and his world. Health and welfare services relevant to the past are no longer germane. Nursing carries a signal responsibility in the great task of designing and implementing health and welfare services commensurate with changing times and human needs. Nursing's potential for meaningful human service rests on the union of theory and practice for its fulfillment.

Hopefully the ideas presented in this book will provide a base for extensive critical thinking and for the further elaboration of nursing's scientific system. Validity must be tested and retested in the arena of nursing practice. Only the future can reveal the extent to which these aims may be realized.

Martha E. Rogers

goodwill and ignorant benevolence as bases for nursing practice brought recriminations from many nurses, doctors, and others. In spite of the demonstrable superiority of "Nightingale-trained" nurses, vested interests persevered in their short-sighted efforts to distort and undermine the integrity of developing schools of nursing.

American nursing arose within the framework of the Industrial Revolution, the Victorian era, mushrooming of hospitals, increasing humanitarianism, and the stirrings of the feminist movement. But the establishment of schools of nursing in the United States abrogated a basic premise on which true Nightingale schools were founded, namely: a school of nursing must be autonomous and clearly separate from service agencies. The historical accident that placed schools of nursing in America under hospital control is only now being rectified. Despite the handicap of unsound governance, leaders in nursing arose whose vision and unwavering vigilance brought about constructive movement. By the end of the nineteenth century, organized nursing was a reality. Vital and imaginative concern for man's well-being was evidenced by initiation in 1901 by the Instructive Nursing Association of Boston of the first prenatal care to be offered by any group in America. Social responsibility soon became evident in licensing laws for protection of the public.

In the past fifty years there have been two World Wars. Conflicting ideologies continue to threaten an uneasy peace. Multiplying scientific knowledge and sweeping technological advances, growing interdependency among nations, and changing concepts of man's responsibility to man characterize the contemporary scene. With man's advent into outer space, the future dimensions of his world stretch beyond imagination. Rapidly accumulating data are forcing new explanations of life and its relation to the universe. Roles and responsibilities of health personnel relevant to the past are no longer relevant for the future. Nursing is in a rapid state of transition.

Nursing's concern for human beings is greater today than it has ever been, because knowledge brings with it increased capacity for meaningful service. The potential of nursing for contributing to human health and welfare has taken on new dimensions. The emergence of professionally educated men and women from the nation's colleges and universities, possessing the substantial scientific knowledge indispensable to safe nursing services in today's world, is an event of major proportions. No longer can experience be equated with learning. Technical and vocational education are fragile products, dangerously applied without knowledgeable leadership. Intellectual skill in utilizing nursing's body of scientific knowledge is a determining factor in professional nursing practice.

An organized body of scientific knowledge—nursing science—is only now assuming identifiable shape. Principles that describe, explain, and predict human behavior, integral to nursing, are emerging. The art of nursing is taking on new dimensions of artistry as it becomes underwritten with its own body of scholarly knowledge. Tomorrow's nurses will be as different from today's as today's are from those of ages past.

The student who selects nursing today has two careers from which to choose: professional or technical. This book is written for those students who have embarked upon a professional career in nursing. It is designed to introduce students to the theoretical basis of professional practice in nursing. Its mission is the transmission of a body of scholarly knowledge that can be translated into human service.

This book is about people: how they are born, and live, and die; in health and in sickness; in joy and in sorrow. It is a story of changing times and new knowledge. The past and future join hands as students are helped to understand the basic concepts of man's evolution and his march toward self-fulfillment. Man's biological, physical, social, psychological, and spiritual heritages become an indivisible whole as scientific facts are merged with human warmth. Better health for mankind is its goal.

The revolution that brought modern nursing into being laid the foundation for today's sweeping changes. For those who seek nursing's knowledge for service to man, there lies a vast, unexplored range of possibilities. The students of today stand on the threshold of a new and expanding era in fulfilling the ages-old commitment of nursing to human health and welfare.

FOOTNOTES

1. Seymer, Lucy R., *A General History of Nursing*, New York: The Macmillan Co., 1939, p. 30.

BACK OF MODERN NURSING

UNIT 1

"Is there such a thing as an impartial history? And what is history? The written representation of past events. But what is an event . . . It is a notable fact. Now, how is the historian to discriminate between whether a fact is notable or no? He decides this arbitrarily, according to his character and idiosyncracy, at his own taste and fancy . . . in a word, as an artist . . ."

—Anatole France
The Garden of Epicuras

needles have been found, mute testimony that Paleolithic man wore clothes, though what the styles of those times may have been is unknown. Art forms, of startling excellence by any standards, were in abundance. Paintings, sculptures, and engravings speak of magic, with hunting and fertility predominant themes. One might suspect that the expertly sculptured handles of utensils may have been a source of pride to many of the tribal women. Marriage regulations and burial rites were followed. Nature gods and tribal ancestors appeared. The latter were perceptive people with highly developed artistic and aesthetic senses.

The Upper Paleolithic period was succeeded by the Mesolithic (12,000 B.C. to 7000 B.C.). The bow and arrow had clearly been invented. Men fished with hook and line. The canoe came into existence. The world's waterways were a source of food and transportation. Animals were domesticated, particularly dogs. Improved tools made tree felling possible. Elementary pottery, baskets, and pebbles painted with mysterious designs marked man's growing mind. Memory and intellectual abstractions, a sense of values and spiritual phenomena, were readying man for his next development.

The Neolithic Age (7000 B.C. to 3000 B.C.) marked such a change in the ways of man that it is often called the Neolithic Revolution. *People began to grow food, not just gather it.* Farming villages appeared. Cattle, goats, sheep, pigs, and dogs became part of the communal life. The potter's wheel (probably preceding the wagon wheel) was used to make bowls, jars, and other items. Spinning and weaving were known. Linen cloth was made from flax. Astronomical computations and predictions were sophisticated and amazingly accurate. Engineering feats of mammoth proportions are evident in huge, rough stone monuments with pillars, archways, and chambers. People led a more settled life. Groups of powerful gods, derived from nature and formed into a sort of family, had to be worshiped and propitiated. Life was hedged with multiple taboos and complicated magic. Wisdom and power were vested in the religious leaders and the elders of the tribes.

The advent of agriculture brought more leisure. Science, art, and religion combined to provide new inventions, more elaborate art work, and growing awareness of one's fellow men. No longer did mothers have to kill their young at birth because they could care for no more children in their nomadic wanderings. Populations began to expand. Simultaneously, around this planet, primitive culture was finding expression. Houses of timber, mud-plastered walls, thatched roofs, and wooden floors made life more comfortable.

People wore simple clothes, probably loose garments. Perhaps shawls were worn over one shoulder and under the other. They painted designs on their skin (how like the modern female!). Male and female roles were more clearly differentiated. No doubt the women of those times were developing a growing pharmacopoeia of useful remedies for care of the sick and injured. Though belief in fickle spirits and cosmic terrors laid heavy prohibitions on all facets of primitive life, empirical knowledge in the rich resources of nature provided practical treatments for a multitude of ills.

One's name was a vital portion of oneself. Newborn infants were frequently given names of powerful or obnoxious animals to ward off demons who might harm them. Great secrecy about one's name was often practiced as a means of protection from mischievous and dangerous spirits.

The universe revolved about man, transcended only by his gods. He had survived centuries of hardship and catastrophic events. Domination by brawn had succumbed to domination by brain. And as the Neolithic period drew to a close, man stood on the threshold of new inventions that would again revolutionize his future. Ancient civilizations were in the offing. Copper and bronze would soon decorate the temples and give new expression to man's ingenuity. A written language would bear testimony to man's evolving nature, his social and cultural developments, his growing science and technology, and a refashioned fabric of philosophy and religion.

No clear-cut date separates the Neolithic period from the rise of civilizations. Unevenness in cultural and scientific developments characterized the peoples of the earth. Quite probably civilized man is much older than we think. But the age of written history had arrived.

FOOTNOTES

1. *New York Times*, Saturday, November 7, 1964.
2. *Nursing Science*, Vol. 2, No. 5, October, 1964, p. 427.
3. *Scientific American*, 212 (5) :50-51, May, 1965.
4. Huxley, Thomas H., *Man's Place in Nature*, Ann Arbor, Michigan: The University of Michigan Press, 1959, p. 184. (Originally published under the title *Evidence as to Man's Place in Nature*, January, 1863.)

CHAPTER 2

MAN'S DEVELOPING CULTURE

". . . the very meaning of human life lies in the fulfillment of values and purposes that issue out of past continuities and are directed toward an ever developing future."

—Lewis Mumford

More than 5,000 years ago in the land of Babylon, there flourished a civilization whose religious and spiritual concepts profoundly influenced nearly all the peoples of the Near East including the Hebrews and Greeks, and ultimately permeated the modern civilized world. The great civilizations of Egypt, Mesopotamia, Persia, and others are indebted to the Sumerians for their basic law, religion, science, and literature. These peoples had a highly developed economic, political, and social structure. They bequeathed a vast and beautiful literature, largely poetry, to subsequent peoples. Epics, myths, lamentations, hymns, proverbs, and words of wisdom testify to man's rich heritage of mind and spirit.

The cuneiform method of writing was invented by the people of Sumer. They also provided the first written record describing man-made subdivisions of the years, months, and days (c. 3500 B.C.). Their ideal year was 12 months of 30 days each, with each day subdivided into 12 danna (roughly equal to two modern hours).[1]

The Sumerian myth of creation explains the origin of the universe as beginning with the primeval sea. The primeval sea begot the cosmic mountain consisting of heaven and earth united. The gods were given human form; An (heaven) was the male and Ki (Earth) the female. They begot the air-god, Enlil, who separated heaven from earth. An carried off heaven and Enlil carried off his mother, Ki, the earth. It was Enlil who "caused the good day to come forth"; who set his mind to "bring forth seed from the earth" and to establish plenty, abundance, and prosperity in the land.[2] Theirs was a polytheistic faith with sun, moon, stars, planets, water, air, grain, etc., each possessing its own appropriate god or goddess. Another legend describes Gilgamesh (great Sumerian hero and forerunner of the Greek Heracles) slaying the snake "who knows no charm" and goes on to discuss the dangers of the "nether world."

Most ancient mythologies give the earth a liquid origin. Egyptian and Hebrew writings reflect this concept. In Polynesia there is a legend that the god Tangora fished up the world from the ocean, but that his line broke and only those pieces known as the South Sea Islands remained above the waves.

The developmental phases of man's cultural evolution followed a similar sequence of events in the various sectors of the planet, with advancements apparently appearing independently (although unevenly in time) among widely separated populations.

Ancient civilizations arose and prospered in the river valleys and irrigated lands. For 2,500 years (3000 B.C. to 525 B.C.) Egypt had a single civilization of remarkable stability. Stylus and papyrus provided a simpler means of recording man's transactions and the story of his life than did the cumbersome cuneiform method developed by the Sumerians. Mathematics and astronomy flourished. Architectural and engineering achievements of great beauty and precision came into being.

The land of the Pharaohs also produced the world's first known genius of historic times. Imhotep, Vizier to King Djoser in the third dynasty, became celebrated as an astronomer, architect, writer, sage, and physician. He produced the vast monument we know today as the Step Pyramid. Egypt's cult of the dead and her yet unsurpassed process of embalming furthered the extraordinary development of medicine and surgery. But mistakes were costly. The Babylonian Legal Code (Code of Hammurabi—about 1900 B.C.) states that "surgeons making successful incisions should be paid in silver, but should have their hands cut off if they caused the death of their patients."

Concern about growing old appears in the Papyrus Smith (c. 3000 to 2500 B.C.) in a "Recipe for Transforming an Old Man into a Youth." A paste, to be kept in a container of semiprecious stones, was prepared and the following instructions given for its usage:

Anoint a man therewith. It is a remover of 'wrinkles' from the head. When the flesh is smeared therewith, it becomes a beautifier of the skin, a remover of 'blemishes,' of all 'weaknesses' which are in the flesh. Found effective myriads of times. (J. H. Breasted, Transl., *The Edwin Smith surgical papyrus*, Vol. 1, p. 498. Chicago: University of Chicago Press, 1930.)[3]

Socially reprehensible behavior is reflected in the ancient Egyptian Declaration of Innocence, for example:

I have not defrauded the oppressed one of his property; I have not done that which is an abomination to the gods; I have not defrauded the temples of their offerings; I have not driven off the cattle from the property of the gods . . . I have not done evil to mankind; I have not caused pain; I have done no murder, nor ordered murder to be done by others.[4]

Contemporary with ancient Egypt was a long-forgotten empire which developed in the Indus Valley of western India. For a thousand years (c. 2500 B.C. to 1500 B.C.) the Harappa people thrived and then somehow disappeared. The two Indus cities were laid out with mathematical precision. Houses were of fired brick with inside baths and emptying ducts to the outside. Interior walls were plastered. The Harappas possessed a fully developed script quite unlike that of the Sumerians.

Thirty-five hundred years ago Stone Age men in what is now Britain were constructing an astronomical observatory of amazing complexity, known today as Stonehenge.[5] Its designers were excellent astronomers, quite conversant with the lunar cycles, and competent in the art of prediction.

Parallel civilizations appeared in India, China, Persia, Mesopotamia, Central America, and other places.

Catastrophic events punctuated man's existence. The Biblical Flood was attributed by William Whiston (successor to Newton at Cambridge) to "the gravitational by-product of a passing comet, which drew up all the waters from the surface of the earth and submerged the dry land."[6] Though Whiston's theory was deemed quite ridiculous by his scientific peers, he is not alone in suggesting that a passing comet may have had major effects on this planet.

In the days of Moses and Joshua (c. 1500 B.C.), there was a great upheaval. Rocks fell from the sky. The waters piled up in immense tides. Fire rained upon the earth and the rivers ran with blood. The earth quaked and the sun stood still. As the records of civilizations have been unearthed, they document castastrophes of like description around the planet, parallel in time. In 1950 Immanuel Velikovsky,[7] scholar and scientist, proposed that Venus was then a comet that had run amok, causing enormous cataclysms. Earth was caught deep in the tail of the comet. Only later would Venus become a planet. Chaos was severe. Moreover, history records more than one world-wide cosmic catastrophe. Velikovsky, with massive documentation and consummate literary skill, reconstructed multiple previously unexplained events. His arguments are cogent. So far his theories have stood the test of time, of a Venus probe, and of increasingly sophisticated astronomical and space research. Did a comet create a South African gold field? Was the legendary continent of Atlantis lost beneath the waves in an upheaval attending a Venus-Earth collision? Did the planet Mars have gases stripped away as it too crossed the path of the errant Venus? How immutable are the orbits of celestial bodies?

Hebrew culture gave to Western man (and also to Islam) a monotheistic faith. Though early Hebrew stories of creation and Biblical references to man's origin are indistinguishable from many of those which appear in Near Eastern cosmology, the concept of one all-powerful God was a signal departure from earlier beliefs. Later, Christianity would adopt the Old Testament as its own.

Hebrew monotheism was not carried over into Greek culture. However, aside from the Greek gods, Western civilization is a continuation of Greek philosophy, politics, government, humanism, and other facets of Greek life. The Greeks were great innovators. Their typical political and social unit was the city-state. Democracies developed. Philosophers, poets, statesmen, mathematicians, and scientists added substantially to the growing world of knowledge and ideas. Theorizing was added to description.

Men sought the basic substance of which all things are made. Three men of Miletus (6th century B.C.) set forth their respective claims. Thales believed it was a clear liquid. Anaximenes said it was a colorless gas. Anaximander thought it was some boundless and imperishable substance.

The quest for a single unifying principle that would explain the nature of life itself engaged these early scientists and philosophers. Heraclitus of Ephasus proposed that the essential condition of life was change. Lucippus and Democritus postulated tiny finite substances called atoms. Pythagoras believed that it was not a substance but a harmonious system of numbers that ordered the universe.

The first known nongeocentric theory of the universe was proposed by the Pythagoreans. The sun and planets were said to revolve around a "central fire." Anaximander produced a theory of evolution, and Empedacles of Sicily held that attraction and repulsion were behind the combination of elements. A concept of man integral to his environment appears in the Hippocratic writings:

> ... health depends upon a state of equilibrium among the various internal factors which govern the operations of the body and the mind; this equilibrium in turn is reached only when man lives in harmony with his external environment.

The great libraries of Alexandria and the numerous astronomical observations of the Mesopotamian priests provided a base from which to formulate theories. The earth was described as spherical in shape, and Aristarchus, though he had few supporters, claimed that the earth circled the sun.

Greek religion is generally described as anthropomorphic (the attributing of human shape and characteristics to the gods). Nor were the Greek gods necessarily immortal. The early Greeks left a rich legacy of myths and legends. Taboos, carried over from prehistoric times, appear. For example, generally iron could not be brought into Greek sanctuaries. Demeter, wife of Zeus and mother of Persephone, was sometimes called "Nurse of the Cornstalks," symbolizing a fertility theme of long standing.

Classical Greek art and architecture remain today, expressions of seldom-equaled beauty, harmony, and imagination.

The establishment and growth of the Roman Republic paralleled in much of time the development of Greek culture. In general it was ruled by a few men of wealth, with the patricians holding a monopoly of public office. Domestic reforms of modern-day equivalence were instigated by Caesar when he returned to Rome as sole dictator in 45 B.C. A census was taken, free grain was distributed to those who needed and deserved it, colonization projects were begun, a public-works program including road construction was instituted, and a system of regular annual taxes was established. The Roman Empire emerged.

The rise of Christianity marked a new period in man's development. By the beginning of the 4th century it was already the most
important religion in the Roman Empire. By the end of the same
century the emperor, Theodosius, proclaimed it their sole religion.
Christians were called upon to aid in the conquest of other peoples
and nations. The Crusades began. With the success of the first
Crusade, papal prestige advanced, later to recede as religious motivation for the warring practices diminished. Nonetheless the emerging medieval world was dominated by the Church. Theology was
central in the rise of the universities. The rediscovery of Aristotle's
writings stifled thinking and at the same time created conflict in
the widely held beliefs of that day. With sophisticated logic Thomas
Aquinas sought to reconcile the two and convinced the Church
authorities that they were not incompatible.

The Dark Ages (14th and 15th centuries) symbolized a decline
in religious, cultural, and political life. For 200 years few innovations appeared in the Western World. However, those that did
presaged the beginnings of modern science. The end of this period
is marked by the revolutionary discoveries of Copernicus (1473-1543)
and Galileo (1564-1642). Movable type was developed by Johann
Gutenberg. Traditional beliefs were overthrown (though not without a desperate struggle) as the concept of a heliocentric world became underwritten with indisputable evidence. The age of discovery
was born.

Commercial enterprise, world-wide in scope, engaged many
peoples. Colonization of the New World, discovered by Columbus,
grew. Italian intellectuals initiated the "cult of antiquity." Religious wars sprang up in opposition to the Church's growing mer-
cantilism, heavy taxes, and brutal treatment of dissident clergymen
and proponents of heretical ideas. The Protestant Reformation was
under way. Andreas Vesalius, Professor at the University of Padua,
was founding anatomy as a science. By 1700 the first stirrings of the
Industrial Revolution were felt, spurred on by a changing political
philosophy engendered by Rousseau, Hume, and Voltaire. The
breakdown of medieval philosophy was in progress.

". . . more than any other figure in the seventeenth century,
Descartes marks the transition from the Middle Ages to the modern
world."[8] Science, philosophy, and religion, as well as government,
politics, and human values, were taking on radically new dimensions. Renewed efforts to explain man and the world he lived in

would soon produce major but clearly dichotomous points of view which were to have a great influence on man's ways of thinking about himself.

FOOTNOTES

1. Dangin, F. Thureau, *Equisse d'une Histoire Sexagesimal,* Paris: P. Geuthner, 1932.

2. Kramer, Samuel Noah, *Sumerian Mythology,* New York: Harper and Brothers, 1961, p. 40.

3. Grant, Richard L., "Concepts of Aging: An Historical Review," *Perspectives in Biology and Medicine,* The University of Chicago Press, Vol. VI, No. 4, summer, 1963, pp. 443-478.

4. Easton, Stewart C., *A Survey of Ancient, Medieval, and Modern History,* New York: Barnes and Noble, Inc., 1964, p. 14.

5. Hawkins, Gerald, *Stonehenge Decoded,* Garden City, N. Y.: Doubleday & Co., Inc., 1965.

6. Toulmin, S. and Goodfield, J., *The Discovery of Time,* New York: Harper Torchbooks, 1965, pp. 94-95.

7. Velikovsky, Immanuel, *Worlds In Collision,* Garden City, N. Y.: Doubleday & Co., Inc., 1950.

8. Eaton, R. M., *Descartes Selections,* New York: Charles Scribner's Sons, 1927. Introduction, p. v.

CHAPTER **3**

THE RISE OF MODERN SCIENCE

"Scientific knowledge is a body of statements of varying degrees of certainty—some most unsure, some
nearly sure, none absolutely certain."

—Richard Feynman

The foundations of modern science were clearly evident in the seventeenth century. William Harvey (1578-1657) discovered the circulation of the blood. Blaise Pascal (1623-1662) invented the theory of probability and measured atmospheric pressure. Robert Boyle (1627-1691) described the relation between the pressure and the volume of a gas. Johannes Kepler (1571-1630) drew his epoch-making conclusions that all the planets moved, not in circles, but in ellipses around the sun, illustrating well the thread of continuity between past inquiry and new knowledge. Calling Tycho Brahe (1546-1601) the "Phoenix of astronomers," Kepler found in Brahe's work observations and measurements of such accuracy and abundance as to provide the foundation for Kepler's investigations. Nor were these the only geniuses in the growing world of science.

Ideas mushroomed in the intoxicating climate of discovery. Each new disclosure led to further searches after truth. Bridging the seventeenth and eighteenth centuries, Sir Isaac Newton (1642-1727) formulated his laws of motion and gravitation. Later Whitehead was to note that the work of Galileo, Newton, Descartes and Huygens (1629-1695) "has some right to be considered as the greatest single intellectual success which mankind has achieved."[1] Oxygen was discovered by an Englishman, Joseph Priestley (1733-1804), and by a Frenchman, Antoine Lavoisier (1743-1794). A system for classifying plants and animals was developed by a Swedish botanist, Carolus Linnaeus (1743-1794); this system is still in use today.

The fine arts, too, found eminent expression in the great wave of creativity sweeping England and the Continent. The portraits of

Rubens (1577-1640) and Rembrandt (1606-1669) left their indelible mark on man's spirit. Baroque music found exquisite distinction in the works of Handel (1685-1759) and Johann Sebastian Bach (1685-1750). Mozart (1756-1791), Beethoven (1770-1827), and Chopin (1810-1849), in turn, gave the world magnificient measures of rapturous melody, depth of feeling, and the spirit of romanticism. John Milton's (1608-1674) poetry stirred men's souls with its rolling tones and majestic visions. Molière's (1622-1673) comedies brought laughter and the tragedies of Racine (1639-1699) drew tears. The Western world moved through the baroque, the rococo, and the romantic.

Philosophy in the latter part of the sixteenth century was deeply imbued with an understanding of the nature of the universe in the medieval tradition. This doctrine made broad claims to the "as above, so below" concept whereby religious beliefs and ideas of the physical universe were seen to be complementary. Consequently, the philosophy of the day was strongly impregnated by a need to accept only those interpretations of physical findings which would also give credence to religious dogma. This led to rigid ritualization of thought through which the safety of compromise and circumvention, rather than the challenge of truth, was the prize.

Nonetheless, by the close of the sixteenth century there was to appear a growing pessimism in religious thought and a spreading skepticism of intellectual ideas. The central figure who set in motion the changing mood of the Western world was René Descartes (1596-1650). Descartes was determined to do away with all the teaching of the ancient world, to doubt everything, and to begin anew in his attempt to explain all aspects of nature according to a single system of principles. Singlehanded, Descartes evolved a natural philosophy that continues to influence modern thought.

It is recorded[2] that Descartes had a startling revelation one night which was to guide his thoughts so forcibly that he remembered the date, November 10, 1619, to the end of his life. This striking disclosure revealed that the key to the mysteries of the universe was in its mathematical order. Consequently, it was in rational and deductive formulations that Descartes founded what became, in effect, the basis of a modern philosophy which considers these two to be the only means of eliminating error to a chance factor in the pursuit of knowledge.

Descartes was much impressed by the achievements of the natural science which came to be known as physics. He determined that his theories would include no mental or spiritual terms, not only with reference to the planets and other physical phenomena but also in his explanations of animal activities and bodily processes in humans. Animals he confidently viewed as machines. However, harking back to his own obeisance to the Church, he played havoc with his sytem of logic when he considered man. Cartesian dualism was born. "Mind" and "matter" were noted to be two fundamentally distinct "substances." As it happens, even animal behavior cannot be categorized into two distinct "substances." It should not be so surprising, then, that scientists who followed Descartes would carry the mechanistic approach further and conclude that man, too, was a machine that could be explained by physical laws. "Around 1700, the sciences of matter, life, and mind reached a parting of the ways. Chemistry, physiology and psychology went off in three separate directions."[3]

Descartes saw man as lord over the forces of nature and endowed with free will. At the same time, when it came to considering the ways in which man obtained knowledge and verified his findings, Descartes joined with Plato, who clearly recognized the difference between scientific fact (episteme) and mere opinion (doxa). According to Plato: "We must concern ourselves with nothing but the objects about which our mind seems capable of acquiring knowledge both certain and indubitable,"[4] thereby enunciating the limitations which humanness imposes upon man. In this manner Descartes rejected human intuition as anything but a rational operation in which particular truths were self-evident, much as were axioms in mathematics. This naive conception of intuition was later to be refuted by such thinkers as Jeans,[5] who indicated that certain mathematical constructs, arithmetic for example, are conditioned by particular assumptions upon which the meaning of integer is based. In Jeans's example certain arithmetical theorems do not hold. For instance, drops of water on a windowpane will upon occasion merge into one, rather than behave as an arithmetic progression. Perhaps Descartes could not have avoided this naiveté without anticipating the findings of Isaac Newton.

Newton's works, which were published late in Descartes' life, were based in the uncommon sense of calculus. Newton invented the calculus for counting hours and measuring angles which accounted for seemingly weird equalities $12 + 1 = 1$ and $360 + 1 = 1$.[6] Descartes' most famous axiom, that two things equal to a third thing are equal to each other, was invalidated shortly after his death by the popular development of the microscope, which elicited deviations in the structure of organisms which had never been apparent to the naked eye. Nevertheless, the brilliance of Descartes' grasp of mathematical concepts was such that his philosophy was upheld as classic through the years.

Descartes, with Pierre de Fermat, developed one of the most powerful innovations in mathematics, that of analytic geometry. This is in actuality an algebraic representation of geometry which is analytic in a particular way. It considers the unknown (x) as if it were, in fact, known and then works back by specified and controlled manipulations of equations. This provided what Hawkins[7] has called a "dictionary by which geometrical problems could be translated into algebraic ones." It should be noted, however, that this methodology—analysis—is antithetic to that of synthesis, which is a genuine process of discovery, even though Descartes' analytic geometry eliminated the ancient requirement for the ruler and the compass in the solution of geometrical problems.

Similarly, Descartes introduced, together with Thomas Hobbes, the unifying concept of cause and effect which was instrumental in integrating the far-flung and highly specialized knowledges of the mid-seventeenth century. Together with Newton, who showed cause even in celestial orbits, they helped to revise the entire concept of natural law by replacing the idea of the human will as directing agent with concepts of cause and of force.[8]

During Descartes' lifetime two societies were founded to pioneer the critical thought which stormed the bulwarks of meaningless medieval tautologies and formed the bridge over which fundamental changes in the subsequent scientific revolution were wrought. The Academie Royale of France and the Royal Society of England came into existence.

At the same time that Descartes was developing the deductive system as the clearly necessary means for discovering truth, Francis Bacon (1561-1626) was emphasizing the method of induction. Cartesian reasoning from the known to the unknown, from the general to the specific, found a ready opponent in Bacon, who believed that one properly moved from the particular to the general. Bacon stressed the need for substantial experimentation in scientific study.

But in the seventeenth century Cartesian thinking dominated the scientific world. Not until the eighteenth and nineteenth centuries did Baconian logic move into a prominent place in man's critical examination of his world. And not until the twentieth century did man come to recognize the value of both methods to scientific study.

Bacon stressed, above all, the need for well-organized experiments to replace the ill-conceived, haphazard investigations of his times. He insisted that experiments be recorded. From experiments one should be able to draw generalizations that will then point the way to further experiments. He remarked that some of those things which are so familiar as to seem self-evident were most in need of study.

Bacon believed that science should transcend the ordinary world of commonsense phenomena. Generalizations too close to concrete facts had little use. Concomitantly, he placed the highest generalizations as out of reach, too near to God and to final causes. These he proposed should be dealt with by the philosophers.

Despite growing emphasis on man as a machine, there were also those who sought an explanation for those behaviors in living things which could not be accounted for within the confines of chemistry and physics. The presence of a subtle, nonmaterial essence, different from and superior to physical matter, was postulated. A vital principle was proposed to differentiate the living from the nonliving.

Vitalism, as it is called, made its major contribution in indicating that the fundamentals of life required more than physicochemical laws for their elucidation. However, the "vital spirit" could not stand up to rigorous, hard-core, scientific study. It could not be caught in a test tube, and its immaterial nature provided little basis for identifying its supposedly causal nature. Around 1770 the anatomist John Hunter proposed an analogy between vitalism and gravity, a comparison which enamored many and which by 1800 had become a refrain in the writings of the physiologists.[9]

Hans Driesch (1867-1941), one of the early experimenters in embryonic development, thought he had an answer to the mechanists in his classic experiment with the beginning phases of the blastula of the sea urchin. Shortly after the first cleavage pinches through the animal-vegetal axis which connects the two poles of the egg, Driesch divided the specimen, cutting directly down the axis. Contrary to his expectation that only nonviable half urchins would result from the two parts, there developed two fully formed organisms which went on to emerge as whole sea urchins. He then concluded that life processes operated by other than physico-chemical laws and that these activities were carried out as though in anticipation of a goal whose meaning was intrinsic. Driesch called this concept "entelechy" and meant to imply thereby that there is purpose to life processes.

Driesch, and others who followed, were greatly impressed by the embryo as an *equipotential system*, that is, every part could produce a complete organism. However, by his experiment, Driesch noted the importance of time in the determination of an embryo's fate, which became progressively more fixed and finally could not be induced to change certain critical factors of development after particular stages of maturity were reached. Nevertheless, purposive-ness of the organism and the species could not be denied in acts of self-preservation and function.

By the mid-eighteenth century man was experiencing a grow-ing unrest. Revolutionary events were taking place in agriculture and industry. Machine technology, mass production, and the steam engine presented problems of great magnitude in government, poli-tics, economics, and employment. The working classes were de-manding benefits and reforms. Numerous utopian schemes were proposed and efforts were made to implement them. Peoples and nations sought independence from the restraining yokes of the power structure. The conflict between science and religion was still powerful, though the static view of nature was beginning to be undermined by emerging knowledge.

FOOTNOTES

1. Whitehead, Alfred North, *Science and the Modern World*, New York: The Macmillan Company, 1926.
2. Bronowski, J., *Common Sense of Science*, New York: Random House, 1953, p. 34.
3. Toulmin, S. and Goodfield, J., *The Architecture of Matter*, New York: Harper Torchbooks, 1966, p. 169.
4. Bunge, Mario, *Intuition and Science*, Englewood Cliffs, New Jersey: Prentice-Hall, Inc., 1962, p. 3.
5. Margenau, Henry, *Open Vistas*, New Haven: Yale University Press, 1961, p. 64.
6. Bunge, *op. cit.*, p. 4.
7. Hawkins, David, *The Language of Nature*, San Francisco: W. H. Free-man and Co., 1964, p. 56.
8. Bronowski, *op. cit.*, p. 95.
9. Toulmin, S. and Goodfield, J., *op. cit.*, p. 324.

CHAPTER **4**

EVOLUTIONARY THOUGHT

"Thoughtful men, once escaped from the blinding influences of traditional prejudice, will find in the lowly stock whence Man has sprung the best evidence of the splendor of his capacities, and will discover in his long progress through the Past reasonable ground of faith in his attainment of a nobler Future."

—Thomas H. Huxley

The nineteenth century saw man's traditional place in nature overthrown. An English naturalist, Charles Darwin (1809-1882), proposed and documented a theory of evolution by natural selection that threatened religious and social upheaval. Publication of Darwin's *On the Origin of the Species* in 1859 stimulated bitter and unbelieving controversy. And even as evidence mounted in support of the theory of evolution, large numbers of people clung tenaciously to literal Biblical interpretations of man's origin. In some of the United States, laws were passed forbidding its instruction. The famous Scopes Evolution Trial in 1925 is late evidence of resistance to evolutionary theory.

Religious opponents of Darwin's theory were vocal and abusive. Misinterpretations were rife. Numerous tracts were written and sermons preached by vehement reactors. An element of humor was inserted when it was reported that "when the Bishop of Worcester communicated the intelligence to his wife that the horrid Professor Huxley had announced that man was descended from the apes, she exclaimed: 'Descended from the apes! My dear, let us hope that it is not true, but if it is, let us pray that it will not become generally known.' "[1] But alas for the Bishop's wife. Not only has the theory of evolution become well known, but it has had a massive influence on contemporary thought.

That Darwin's theory should have had an almost instantaneous impact on religion, science, and the general public should not be

23

surprising. Herbert Spencer (1820-1903) had already coined the phrase "survival of the fittest" before Darwin's book was published. Thomas R. Malthus (1766-1834) had laid a foundation for a concept of natural selection in his works on human population. Malthus had proposed that populations tend to increase faster than the food supply. Consequently, unless births are controlled, poverty, war, and pestilence must serve as natural restrictions to maintain a state of balance between the numbers of people and the available food supply. Inroads on traditional thinking were already in progress as a result of the work of paleontologists, archeologists, biologists, and anthropologists. Alfred Russel Wallace, working independently, arrived at a comparable theory of evolution almost simultaneously with Darwin.

Perhaps a significant factor in the rapid spread of evolutionary theory lay in the orientation of mid-nineteenth century man to the idea of "progress." Evolution provided a way of conceiving man's potential for advancement. It was used to signify "improvement," a "going forward." Concomitantly, it was used to justify toleration of deplorable social conditions as inevitable evidence of the "survival of the fittest" concept.

Though theologians were generally the first to respond to the impact of change in viewing the origin of man, the implications of evolution cut a broad swath across man's multi-faceted existence. A biologically oriented philosophy was stimulated and supported. Man's place in nature no longer had the fixity associated with earlier theology. Opponents of Darwinism were forced to reconcile their views with evolutionary thought.

Darwin was exceedingly aware of the turmoil he was creating in the minds of men. But the evidence of biological unfolding was so indisputable as to demand recognition. Concomitantly, Darwin realized that the data he had gathered were only a beginning. He stressed the need for research into the causes and laws of variation. He emphasized the pursuit of further understanding of the phenomenon of man's heritage.

At the same time that *On the Origin of the Species* was rocking England, Europe, and America, a quiet Austrian monk, Gregor Mendel (1822-1884), was studying the transmission of hereditary traits by means of extensive experiments with sweet peas. Reports of Mendel's work were available in published form from 1866 on, but interestingly enough, they were ignored until after his death. When rediscovered, they provided substantial empirical evidence

a new cosmology that will better underwrite the world of man. Old premises are no longer adequate on which to build a future. A concept of man as an indivisible phenomenon is emerging. Study of the life process is beginning to focus on man's unity.

With all man's fears and uncertainties, he is nonetheless striving for a growing humanitarian concern. His values are expanding to place increased emphasis on better ways to serve man's health and welfare. True, these changing values cannot be disassociated from man's struggle for survival. Nor can this shrinking planet fail to reflect the growing complexity of man's knowledge and the integrating aspects of the interdependence of peoples around this globe. The story of the universe is a tale of synthesis: the merging of physical, biological, and cultural phenomena into increasing complexity of organization. Man's evolving capacity for meaningful abstractions foretells unifying concepts of fundamental significance.

For more than a million years man has dwelt upon the earth. His vicissitudes have been many. His search for understanding has been persistent. Promotion of health and maintenance of life have been constant attendants upon his march through time. And always he has sought to add meaning to the life he preserved, through religion, philosophy, science, and the fine arts. Man's awareness of mortality threads throughout his history. Death, a condition of living, has been met with laughter and with scoffing, with futility and with faith, with avoidance and with relief. A growing concern for the preservation of man's humanness is finding expression.

The reality of evolutionary change is explicit. Man's development through time reflects growing complexity of pattern and organization. Modern theories of life, not yet discussed, have their roots in a past possessing fewer definitive facts than now exist. Less well-known ideas than many of those heretofore presented add to the foundation of twentieth century man's pursuit of knowledge and understanding.

FOOTNOTES

1. Montagu, Ashley, "Introduction" to Huxley, Thomas H., *Man's Place in Nature,* Ann Arbor, Michigan: The University of Michigan Press, 1959, p. 3.

2. Rensch, Bernard, *Evolution Above the Species Level,* New York: Columbia University Press, 1960, p. 101.

3. Terry, K. and Tucker, W., "Biologic Effects of Supernovae," *Science,* Vol. 159, No. 3813, January 26, 1968, pp. 421-423.

4. Rensch, *loc. cit.*

5. Shaefer, Karl E., *Man's Dependence on the Earthly Atmosphere,* New York: The Macmillan Company, 1962.

CHAPTER **5**

INTO THE TWENTIETH CENTURY

"Neither physical nature nor life can be understood unless we fuse them together as essential factors in the composition of "really real" things whose interconnections and individual characters constitute the universe."

—Alfred North Whitehead

Over the centuries efforts to explain the many attestations of life have led to multiple concepts and theories. Various attributes of living systems have been noted and described. The ancient Greeks believed that human beings could not be understood unless nature as a whole was understood. They held that man and his world were governed by natural laws. Subsequently, the Dark Ages and later centuries brought with them a concept of man as separate from nature. Not until the late seventeenth century was there again a serious scientific proposal that man might also be controlled by natural laws. Newton introduced his concept of an electromagnetic-like medium governing various properties of both the living and the non-living (proposed in 1675 but not published until 1757).[1]

The rise of modern science with its emphasis on a mechanistic approach and mind-body dualism was a firm denial of man and nature as a single system. Science and religion took separate roads. Philosophy was relegated to a remote corner of man's consciousness. Human life was segmented into a variety of discrete entities to be dealt with by distinctly different groups.

Concomitantly, the introduction of evolutionary theory and the discrediting of the theory of spontaneous generation in the latter half of the nineteenth century cracked the veneer of man's belief in his separate existence. Experimental proof that spontaneous generation did not occur had been provided by Francesco Redi (1626-1697) and published in 1668. Notwithstanding, proponents of autogenesis developed numerous experiments and explanations in support of their ideas. The French Academy of Science offered a prize for convincing evidence that would resolve the question. The award went to Louis Pasteur, who in 1862 published his work in this area and left no room for fault-finding by the skeptical. The theory of spontaneous generation was dealt a mortal blow.

Documentation of the germ theory was a further outgrowth of Pasteur's work. The presence of a specific microorganism was demonstrated to be an essential condition for the development of a specific disease. Koch's postulates* became accepted guidelines for determining disease causation. Hope was born that a specific causal agent would be found for each disease. With such knowledge it was dreamt that man might learn to control the sicknesses that beset him. The concept of single causation loomed large. Diseases were noted to be distinct entities, each having its specific cause requiring only man's ingenuity and hard work to identify it. Health and illness became two clearly different dimensions of biological life, each to be studied in its own way. Man as a unified being moved farther out of sight.

At mid-nineteenth century Florence Nightingale had been saving lives in Scutari with her emphasis on sanitation and humane care. Evidence of the effectiveness of her efforts grew. Despite strong protests, modern nursing was born. The nature of man's environment was proposed to be a significant factor in recovery of health. Extensive statistical data accumulated testifying to the validity of Miss Nightingale's arguments. By the end of the century she was emphasizing that maintenance of health was as important as care of the sick. Nightingale's proposals placed man within the framework of the natural world. His humanness was moving into focus. The foundation for the scope of modern nursing was laid.

The physical, biological, and social sciences—in that order— grew and flourished. New branches sprang forth. Scientists became more and more engrossed in specialization. Facts accumulated. In-

---

* KOCH'S POSTULATES: (Taken from Tabor's Cyclopedic Medical Dictionary, 10th Edition).
1. microorganism in question must appear in lesion at all times;
2. pure cultures must be obtained from it;
3. pure cultures when inoculated into susceptible animals must reproduce the disease or pathological condition; and
4. the organism must be obtained again in pure culture from the inoculated animal.

visible walls rose up between the different fields of study. The exploration of man's separate identities built isolated structures of growing complexity. Not only was man viewed as a thing apart from nature but his very integrity as a functioning whole went almost unnoticed.

The study of biological processes emphasized entities: systems, organs, and cells, rather than organization. The cell came to be viewed as the basic unit of life.

Late in the nineteenth century Sigmund Freud brought exploration of the human mind into sharp focus. Freudian theory began to permeate the Western world. Id, ego, and superego were used to provide a topological personality scheme. Life and death instincts were proposed. A theory of the libido (love) was developed. The field of psychoanalysis had its beginnings with the publication of Freud's book *Studies on Hysteria* (1895). A system of psychopathology and psychotherapy was founded.

As the nineteenth century moved into the twentieth, there occurred a momentous discovery in the world of physics that would later stimulate new ideas in the biological and psychosocial sciences. Classical particle physics was supplemented by field physics. Events of the physical world had a new unity. Moreover, it was pointed out that fields and particles could not be observed simultaneously though both phenomena were required for a complete description of what was taking place.

New ways of perceiving the physical world tumbled forth. In 1905 Einstein's theory of relativity shook the scientific world. The four coordinates of space-time replaced man's three-dimensional universe.

Electricity had become firmly ensconced within the field of physics by the beginning of the nineteenth century. In the ensuing years the electrical nature of nonliving matter had become increasingly well known. Concomitantly, though interest in bioelectric phenomena had persisted from the time of Newton, their study had engaged few investigators. Eighteenth century exponents of electricity in living things had endeavored to find supporting evidence for their theories. Mesmer had termed this strange phenomenon "animal magnetism" (1775) and related it directly to the nervous system of animate forms. Several writers of this period suggested that shocks received from the torpedo fish were electrical in nature. Berthalon, in 1783, published the first experiments giving evidence of the influence of atmospheric electricity on vegetation. Luigi Galvani's (1737-1798) historic work on the interaction of frog's legs and electricity laid the groundwork for later study that would substantiate electricity as a property of protoplasmic systems.

Evidence concerning the electrical nature of living systems accumulated slowly. Then, as man moved into the twentieth century, there appeared a revival of interest in the electrical properties of life. Electrical correlates of growth processes were identified. Results of electrometric studies pointed up the presence of polar and potential differences in living systems. Human beings were noted to be characterized by electrical fields.

Growing evidence of man's electrical properties led to technological innovations of high practical value. Encephalography and cardiography were developed to provide additional indices of brain and heart functioning, respectively.

In 1935 H. S. Burr and F. S. C. Northrop published their historic statement of "The Electro-Dynamic Theory of Life."[2] With substantial documentation and logic they postulated:

> The pattern or organization of any biological system is established by a complex electro-dynamic field, which is in part determined by its atomic physico-chemical components and which in part determines the behavior and orientation of those components. This field is electrical in the physical sense and by its properties it relates the entities of the biological system in a characteristic pattern and is itself in part a result of the existence of those entities. It determines and is determined by the components. More than establishing pattern, it must maintain pattern in the midst of a physico-chemical flux. Therefore, it must regulate and control living things, it must be the mechanism the outcome of whose activity is "wholeness," organization and continuity.

"Like the erstwhile atom in chemistry, the cell (had) lost its prestige as the ultimate unit in biology. Both the atomic and cellular theories (had) become obsolete."[3] An electrical field was replacing the cell as the fundamental unit of biological systems. Living things were characterized by pattern and "wholeness" and subject to natural laws.

At the same time that Burr and Northrup were developing biological field theory, Kurt Lewin[4] was evolving psychological field theory. All behavior, according to Lewin, represented a change of some state of field in a given unit of time. The psychological field was conceived as a single, interdependent whole encompassing a wide range of determinants and treated as a single coherent system. Lewin was careful to point out that recognition of an aggregate of factors associated with an event did not presuppose field theory. Rather, it was necessary to view the field as having its own unique integrity. Lewin's principle of contemporaneity was an essential characteristic of this theory. He asserted that although the life space is continuously modified through time, only the contemporary system can have effect at any given point in time. "Any behavior or any other change in a psychological field depends only upon the psychological field at that time."[5] This principle was not a rejection of man's past and future. The continuity of life was recognized. Its dynamic aspects were perceived. But behavior was proposed to be determined by interaction of the person and the environment at any given point in time according to the state of the person and the environment at that time.

Though many theories bred themselves into the fabrics of the natural and social sciences, concepts of man as more than an aggregate of physical, biological, psychological, sociocultural, and spiritual entities were vague and generally suspect. For decades the barriers between man's separate beings had grown higher as each field of science accumulated its own body of facts and theories. A particular sociologist suggested that man was a summation of six selves (physiological, psychological, logical, metaphysical, moral, sociopolitical), and Jacques Barzun with characteristic humor wondered: "Would the glue hold?"[6]

But awareness of the interrelatedness of knowledge was growing. A wide range of determinants were shown to be associated with man's condition. The concept of single causation faded.

Knowledge about electrical fields mushroomed. Communication theory and feed-back operations began to be used to offer other explanations of human behavior. In 1956 G. D. Wasserman[7] introduced electrical field theory to explain organismic form and behavior. Postulating energy fields in living systems analogous to those postulated in physics, he proposed an electrical field theory to account for morphogenesis, behavior, and parapsychological phenomena.

Space research encompassing multiple facets of human behavior—physical, physiological, psychological, and environmental—initiated vast new areas of conjecture about man's potentials and limitations. Many traditional concepts moved toward obsolescence. New theories came to be formulated and tested.

A description of biological man (or psychological man, etc.) no more describes the human being than a description of hydrogen (or oxygen) describes water. The properties of a living system are clearly different from those of its components. Man is a unified phenomenon subject to natural laws and characterized by a complex electrodynamic field. He is more than and different from the sum of his parts. Physicochemical laws are inadequate to explain him. Feed-back models fail to consider his dynamic, unidirectional, growing complexity. Man's consciousness and creativity are integral dimensions of man's wholeness.

Nursing's age-old commitment to human health and welfare has taken on new dimensions. The fundamental assumptions on which nursing knowledge and nursing practice rest are being rewritten by the very terms of man's existence. People are at the center of nursing's purpose. The descriptive, explanatory, and predictive principles that direct professional nursing practice are rooted in a fundamental concept of the wholeness of life.

FOOTNOTES

1. Ravitz, Leonard J., "Studies of Man in the Life Field," *MAIN CURRENTS in Modern Thought*, Vol. 19, No. 1, September-October, 1962, p. 14.
2. Burr, H. S. and Northrop, F. S. C., "The Electro-Dynamic Theory of Life," *The Quarterly Review of Biology*, 10:322-333, 1935.
3. Morgulis, S., "Introduction to the Second Edition" of Oparin, A. I., *The Origin of Life*, New York: Dover Publications, Inc., 1953, p. xvi.
4. Lewin, Kurt, *Field Theory in Social Science*, edited by Dorwin Cartwright, New York: Harper Torchbooks, 1964.
5. *Ibid.*, p. 45.
6. Barzun, Jacques, *Science: The Glorious Entertainment*, New York: Harper and Row, 1964, p. 306.
7. Wasserman, G. D., "An Outline of a Field Theory of Organismic Form and Behavior," *Extrasensory Perception*, Boston: Little, Brown and Company, 1956, pp. 53-72.

RELATED READINGS

ADLER, MORTIMER J., *The Idea of Freedom*, Garden City, N. Y.: Doubleday & Co., Inc., 1958.

ALDRED, CYRIL, *The Egyptians*, New York: Frederick A. Praeger, Publisher, 1961.

ALLEN, E. L., *From Plato to Nietzsche*, Greenwich, Conn.: Fawcett Publications, Inc., 1957.

ARDREY, ROBERT, *African Genesis*, New York: Atheneum Press, 1961.

ASIMOV, ISAAC, *The Wellspring of Life*, New York: The New American Library, 1960.

———, *Life and Energy*, New York: Doubleday & Co., Inc., 1962.

BARNETT, ANTHONY, *The Human Species*, Baltimore, Md.: Penguin Books, 1957.

BARRETT, WILLIAM, *Irrational Man*, Garden City, N. Y.: Doubleday Anchor Books, 1962.

BARROW, GEORGE, *Your World in Motion*, New York: Harcourt, Brace and World, Inc., 1956.

BARZUN, JACQUES, *Science: The Glorious Entertainment*, New York: Harper and Row, 1964.

BERRILL, N. J., *Man's Emerging Mind*, New York: Fawcett World Library, 1955.

BERTALANFFY, LUDWIG VON, *Problems of Life*, New York: Harper Torchbooks, 1960.

BLUM, HAROLD, *Time's Arrow and Evolution*, New York: Harper Torchbooks, 1962.

BOHR, NIELS, *Atomic Theory and the Description of Nature*, Cambridge: The University Press, 1934.

BONNER, JAMES, *The Molecular Biology of Development*, New York: Oxford University Press, 1965.

BRONOWSKI, J., *Commonsense of Science*, New York: Random House, 1953.

———, *Science and Human Values*, revised edition, New York: Harper Torchbooks, 1965.

BUNGE, MARIO, *Intuition and Science*, Englewood Cliffs, N. J.: Prentice-Hall, Inc., 1962.

BURR, H. S. and LANE, C. T., "Electrical Characteristics of Living Systems," *Yale Journal of Biology and Medicine*, 8:31-35, 1935.

——— and NORTHRUP, F. S. C., "The Electro-Dynamic Theory of Life," *MAIN CURRENTS in Modern Thought*, Vol. 19, No. 1, September-October 1963. pp. 4-10.

BUTTERFIELD, HERBERT, *The Origins of Modern Science*, New York: Collier Books, 1962.

CANNON, WALTER, *The Wisdom of the Body*, New York: W. W. Norton, 1939.

CHAMPION, S. G. and SHORT, D., *Readings from World Religions*, New York: Fawcett World Library, 1959.

COLEMAN, JAMES A., *Modern Theories of the Universe*, New York: The New American Library, 1963.

CROMBIE, A. C., *Medieval and Early Modern Science*, Vol. II, New York: Doubleday & Co., Inc., 1959.

——— (Edit.) , *Turning Points in Physics*, New York: Harper Torchbooks, 1961.

DANTO, A. and MORGANBESSER, S. (Edit.), *Philosophy of Science*, New York: Meridian Books, Inc., 1960.

DEBROGLIE, LOUIS, *The Revolution in Physics*, New York: The Noonday Press, Inc., 1953.

DECHARDIN, TEILHARD, *The Phenomenon of Man*, New York: Harper Torchbooks, 1961.

DEETZ, JAMES, *Invitation to Archaeology*, New York: The Natural History Press, 1967.

DESANTILLANA, GIORGIO, *The Origins of Scientific Thought*, New York: The New American Library, 1961.

DESCARTES, RENÉ, *Meditations*, New York: The Liberal Arts Press, Inc., 1960. (Second Revised Edition.)

DOBZHANSKY, THEODOSIUS, *Mankind Evolving*, New Haven: Yale University Press, 1962.

——, *Evolution, Genetics, and Man*, New York: John Wiley and Sons, Inc., 1963.

——, *Heredity and the Future of Man*, New York: Harcourt, Brace and World, Inc., 1964.

DUNN, L. C., *Heredity and Evolution in Human Populations*, New York: Atheneum Press, 1965.

DUNOÜY, LECOMTE, *Human Destiny*, New York: Longmans, Green and Co., 1947

EASTON, STEWART C., *A Survey of Ancient, Medieval, and Modern History*, New York: Barnes & Noble, Inc., 1964.

EATON, R. M. (Edit.), *Descartes Selections*, New York: Charles Scribner's Sons, 1927.

EINSTEIN, ALBERT, *Relativity*, New York: Crown Publishing Co., Inc., 1961.

EISELEY, LOREN, *The Firmament of Time*, New York: Atheneum Publishers, 1966.

FRANKL, VIKTOR E., *Man's Search for Meaning*, New York: Washington Square Press, Inc., 1963.

FREUD, SIGMUND, *The History of the Psychoanalytic Movement and Other Papers* (with an Introduction by the Editor, Philip Rieff), New York: Collier Books, 1933.

GARDNER, JOHN W., *Excellence*, New York: Harper & Brothers, 1961.

GASTER, THEODOR H., *The New Golden Bough* (a new abridgment of the classic work by Sir James George Frazer), New York: The New American Library, 1959.

GOLDSTEIN, KURT, *The Organism*, New York: The American Book Co., 1939.

GREENE, JOHN C., *Darwin and the Modern World View*, Baton Rouge: Louisiana State University Press, 1961.

HADAS, MOSES, *Humanism*, New York: Harper & Brothers, 1960.

HAGEN, VICTOR VON, *Realm of the Incas*, New York: The New American Library, 1957.

——, *The Aztec: Man and Tribe*, New York: The New American Library, 1958.

HARRISON, JANE ELLEN, *Mythology*, New York: Harcourt, Brace and World, Inc., 1963.

HAVENS, GEORGE R., *The Age of Ideas*, New York: Henry Holt and Co., 1955.

HAWKINS, DAVID, *The Language of Nature*, San Francisco: W. H. Freeman & Co., 1964.

HAWKINS, GERALD, *Stonehenge Decoded*, New York: Doubleday & Co., Inc., 1965.

HEBB, D. O., *The Organization of Behavior*, New York: John Wiley & Sons, Inc., 1949.

HEILBRONER, ROBERT L., *The Worldly Philosophers*, New York: Simon and Schuster, 1961.

HERRICK, C. JUDSON, *The Evolution of Human Nature*, Austin, Texas: The University of Texas Press, 1956.

HOWELLS, WILLIAM, *Back of History*, Garden City, N. Y.: Doubleday & Co., Inc., 1954.

HUXLEY, THOMAS H., *Man's Place in Nature*, Ann Arbor, Mich.: The University of Michigan Press, 1959. (Originally published under the title *Evidence as to Man's Place in Nature*, January 1863.)

JAMES, E. O., *The Ancient Gods*, New York: G. P. Putnam's Sons, 1960.

JEANS, SIR JAMES, *The Growth of Physical Science*, Greenwich, Conn.: Fawcett Publications, Inc., 1961.

JEROME, THOMAS SPENCER, *Aspects of the Study of Roman History*, New York: Capricorn Books, 1962.

JOHNSTON, ARTHUR (Edit.), *Francis Bacon*, New York: Schocken Books, 1965.

KRAMER, SAMUEL NOAH, *Sumerian Mythology*, New York: Harper & Brothers, 1961.

LANGDON-DAVIES, JOHN, *On the Nature of Man*, New York: The New American Library, 1961.

LAWRENCE, WILLIAM L., *New Frontiers of Science*, New York: Bantam Books, 1964.

LEHNINGER, ALBERT L., Bioenergetics, New York: W. A. Benjamin, Inc., 1965.

LEWIN, KURT, *Field Theory in the Social Sciences* (edited by Dorwin Cartwright), New York: Harper Torchbooks, 1964.

LEWINSOHN, RICHARD, *Animals, Men and Myths*, Greenwich, Conn.: Fawcett Publications, Inc., 1954.

LOOMIS, C. P. and LOOMIS, Z. K., *Modern Social Theories*, Princeton, N. J.: D. Van Nostrand Co., 1961.

MARGENAU, HENRY, *Open Vistas*, New Haven: Yale University Press, 1961.

MASON, J. ALDEN, *The Ancient Civilizations of Peru*, Baltimore, Md.: Penguin Books, Inc., 1957.

MEAD, MARGARET (Edit.), *Cultural Patterns and Technical Change*, New York: The New American Library, 1955.

MEDEWAR, P. B., *The Future of Man*, New York: The New American Library, 1961.

METRAUX, GUY S. and CROUZET, FRANCOIS (Edit.), *The Evolution of Science*, New York: The New American Library, 1963.

MUMFORD, LEWIS, *The Transformations of Man*, New York: Harper & Brothers, Publishers, 1956.

———, *The Myth of the Machine*, New York: Harcourt, Brace and World, Inc., 1967.

MURPHY, GARDNER, *Human Potentialities*, New York: Basic Books, Inc., 1958.

NEUMANN, ERICH, *The Origins and History of Consciousness*, New York: Harper Torchbooks, 1962.

NORTHROP, F. S. C., *Man, Nature and God*, New York: Pocket Books, Inc., 1963.

OPARIN, A. I., *The Origin of Life*, New York: Dover Publications, Inc., 1953.

PIEL, GERARD, *Science in the Cause of Man*, New York: Alfred A. Knopf, 1961.

RENSCH, BERNHARD, *Evolution Above the Species Level*, New York: Columbia University Press, 1960.

RUESCH, HANS, *Top of the World*, New York: Pocket Books, Inc., 1951.

RUSSELL, BERTRAND, *The ABC of Relativity*, New York: The New American Library, 1958.

SEARS, PAUL B., *Where There Is Life,* New York: Dell Publishing Co., Inc., 1962.

SEYMER, LUCY R., *A General History of Nursing,* New York: The Macmillan Co., 1939.

—— (Compiled by), *Selected Writings of Florence Nightingale,* New York: The Macmillan Co., 1954.

SHAEFER, KARL E. (Edit.), *Man's Dependence on the Earthly Atmosphere,* New York: The Macmillan Co., 1962.

SHAMOS, MORRIS H. and MURPHY, GEORGE M. (Edit.), *Recent Advances in Science,* New York: Science Editions, Inc., 1961.

SHAPLEY, HARLOW, *The View from a Distant Star,* New York: Dell Publishing Co., a Delta Book, 1964.

SMITH, HOMER W., *From Fish to Philosopher,* New York: Doubleday & Co., Inc., The Natural History Library Edition, 1961.

SPERO, JEANNETTE, "Evolution," *Nursing Science,* Vol. 2, No. 2, April 1964, pp. 139-151.

STACE, W. T., *Religion and the Modern Mind,* Philadelphia: J. B. Lippincott Co., 1952.

SULLIVAN, WALTER, *We Are Not Alone,* New York: McGraw-Hill Book Co., 1964.

THEOBALD, ROBERT, *The Rich and the Poor,* New York: The New American Library, 1961.

THOMAS, ELIZABETH MARSHALL, *The Harmless People,* New York: Alfred A. Knopf, 1959.

THOMPSON, D'ARCY W., *Growth and Form,* second edition, Cambridge: University Press, 1952.

TOCQUET, ROBERT, *Life on the Planets,* New York: Grove Press, Inc., 1962.

TOULMIN, S. and GOODFIELD, J., *The Architecture of Matter,* New York: Harper Torchbooks, 1966.

——, *The Discovery of Time,* New York: Harper Torchbooks, 1966.

TOYNBEE, ARNOLD J., *A Study of History* (abridgement by D. C. Somervell), New York: Oxford University Press, 1947.

——, *Greek Civilization and Character,* New York: The New American Library, 1953.

TRUE, WEBSTER P. (Edit.), *Man and His Works,* New York: Simon and Schuster, Inc. (in cooperation with the Smithsonian Institution, Washington, D. C.), 1960.

VELIKOVSKY, IMMANEL, *Worlds in Collision,* Garden City, N. Y.: Doubleday & Co., Inc., 1950.

WARNER, REX, *The Greek Philosophers,* New York: The New American Library, 1958.

WHITE, MORTON, *The Age of Analysis,* New York: The New American Library, 1955.

WHITEHEAD, ALFRED N., *Science and the Modern World,* New York: The Macmillan Co., 1925.

——, *His Reflections on Man and Nature,* New York: Harper & Brothers, 1961.

THE PHENOMENON OF MAN: NURSING'S CONCERN

UNIT II

"The proper study of mankind is man."
—Alexander Pope

INTRODUCTION TO
UNIT II

Michael Polanyi once wrote: "The existence of animals was not discovered by zoologists, nor that of plants by botanists, and the scientific value of zoology and botany is but an extension of man's pre-scientific interest in animals and plants."* This might be paraphrased to read: "The existence of man was not discovered by nurses, and the scientific value of nursing is but an extension of mankind's continuing efforts to explain man."

Nursing's central concern is with man in his entirety. The process of life and its concomitant, death, are dynamic events of great complexity. The sequential developments of life processes are momentous happenings. A knowledge of life's distinctive characteristics is basic to understanding the multiple manifestations of human behavior.

Human behavior reflects the merging of physical, biological, psychological, social, cultural, and spiritual attributes into an indivisible whole—a whole in which the parts are not distinguishable. Human existence is a unified phenomenon. The distinctive properties of man come into view only as the parts lose their identity. Life's complexity is a haunting melody of continuously interacting variables. The organization and patterning of living systems achieve their greatest complexity in man. Though sharing many attributes in common with other living forms, man possesses a capacity for conscious awareness of himself and the world about him which differentiates him from other life upon this planet. The rudiments of consciousness are transcended and find expression in man's rationality, his capacity for creation, his humanness. People are thinking, feeling beings.

---

* Polanyi, Michael, *Personal Knowledge*, Chicago: The University of Chicago Press, 1958. p. 139.

Nursing's theoretical system is built upon basic assumptions about man. Throughout the remainder of this book the term "man" is used to signify the human being as a single system whose characteristics are identifiably those of the whole.

The study of man encompasses the multiplicity of events that may take place as man moves along the continuum from life through death. Normal and pathological processes are dealt with on a basis of complete equality. Ease and dis-ease are dichotomous notions that cannot be used to account for the dynamic complexity and uncertain fulfillment of man's unfolding.

Unit II is designed to identify and discuss general characteristics of man that are basic to the development and understanding of nursing's unifying principles and hypothetical generalizations which will be taken up in Unit III.

CHAPTER **6**

MAN: A UNIFIED WHOLE

"Whether we are dealing with an atom, galaxy, or a man, the distinctive properties of a whole are significantly different from those of its parts . . ."

—C. Judson Herrick
The Evolution of Human Nature

As has been noted earlier, the ancient Greeks perceived man as a unified being integral to the universe. With the rise of modern science, technological innovations began to produce more and more detailed data about the microscopic and submicroscopic world. Remarkable feats of engineering hatched complex machines purporting to be analogous to human functioning. The unity of man became lost in a plethora of physical and chemical facts. Man came to be explained, not as a human being, but as an operating collection of systems, organs, and cells. Man's sentience was a thing apart from his physical being. Efforts to explore man's mind led to further separation between man's physicophysiological behavior and the phenomenon of consciousness. Only recently has there been growing awareness that man cannot be explained by laws that govern segments of his being.

Steps to bring together the knowledges of several fields can be found in psychology's exploration of the neurological components of emotional behavior. Certain cyberneticists continue to hope that one day they "may be able to explain not only all the functions of the nervous system but also man's total intellectual activity by means of the theory of information or its consequences . . ."[1] Although these efforts reflect growing recognition of the unitary nature of knowledges, they do not provide an understanding of the unitary nature of man.

The unity of man is a reality. Man interacts with his environment in his totality. Only as man's wholeness is perceived does the study of man begin to yield meaningful concepts and theories. Only as man's oneness is apprehended is it possible to identify man's distinctive attributes.

The problem of conceiving man as a whole plagues many people. In spite of frequent protestations of a belief in man's unity, a little probing usually discloses the additive nature of the individual's perception. In recent years attempts to develop unifying theories of human behavior have highlighted basic difficulties in identifying man as a unit of study. Lewis Mumford has noted: "We are too easily tempted today by habits that belong to past moments of civilization, into thinking of the kind of unity that might be achieved by a formal assembly of specialists, by an organization of 'interdisciplinary activities,' by an intellectual synthesis based upon some logical scheme for uniting the sciences."[2] Interdisciplinary discussions have been remarkably limited as a means of arriving at a unified concept of man. Unfortunately the contiguity of persons from a range of fields has generally succeeded in reducing man to the particulars of each field. The whole, then, takes on a chimerical quality inimical to productive inquiry.

As a number of authors have pointed out, the whole cannot be understood when it is reduced to its particulars.[3, 4, 5, 6, 7, 8, 9, 10] With the development of general systems theory, hierarchal systems have been introduced to identify ascending levels of organization as a means of studying living systems. Nor is this approach a new one. In 1862 Virchow[11] proposed that the study of cell, tissue, organism, and social levels must be encompassed by the life sciences.

Miller,[12] in 1965, using general systems behavior theory, distinguished seven levels of living systems (cells, organs, organisms, groups, organizations, societies, and supranational systems) in his development of basic concepts and hypotheses directed toward better understanding the processes of life. Miller[13] further proposed interdisciplinary participation in multilevel research to provide empirical evaluation of his hypotheses. Although Miller pointed out that "more complex systems at higher levels manifest characteristics, more than the sum of the units, not observed at lower levels,"[14] a multisystem approach would seem to perpetuate at least some of the problems inherent in viewing the life process as composed of sets of subsystems and suprasystems and to mitigate against perceiving the wholeness of man.

Edward Purcell has noted that the "most elementary inter-actions can generate, in a large assembly, cooperative behavior the prediction of which challenges our most powerful methods of analysis"[15] and gives a "sober warning to anyone who attempts to carve a path of rigorous deduction from the part to the whole,"[16] whether in physics or in other disciplines.

J. B. Bennett,[17] in a four-volume work entitled *The Dramatic Universe*, endeavors to bring all knowledge into a coherent system and hypothesizes that life has the task of reconciling mechanical and conscious processes throughout the universe. Bennet develops a progession of "categories of fact" and "categories of value." First in his series of "categories of fact" is "wholeness." Wholeness is noted to be omnipresent but relative, and Bennett states: ". . . gradations of wholeness . . . are determined by the extent or degree to which a given object is itself and does not merge into something that is not itself."[18]

Charles Eugene-Guye, a Swiss physicist who died in 1942, stated that "it is the scale of observation which creates the phenomenon."[19] Lecomte duNoüy[20] ably illustrated this statement by pointing out that "the psychology of crowds cannot be deduced from individual psychology." As a further example duNoüy notes that "sodium is a metal, chlorine is a toxic gas, the combination of the two gives sodium chloride, which is harmless kitchen salt. Nothing in the properties of (the sodium and chlorine) atoms enables us to foresee the properties of salt." Knowledge about the subsystems of man, though it may be extensive, is equally ineffective in enabling one to determine the properties of the living system, man.

The properties of man cannot be deduced from the study of biology, physics, psychology, and sociology any more than psychological properties can be deduced from the study of atoms and molecules. While this is not a denial of interactions between subsystems or between levels of organization, it does point up problems that can arise when persons fail to recognize that the properties of the whole are not those of its parts. Nor is intellectual acceptance that man is a system having his own identifiable oneness a guarantee against the common practice of describing man according to one or more subsystems, thereby destroying the meaning of man in his wholeness.

The mind-matter dualism of Cartesian philosophy continues to mitigate against a conception of man's unity. New discoveries in the physical world, coupled with investigations which treat feed-back systems as analogous to human functioning, have encouraged those with leanings toward a mechanistic explanation of life.

Interestingly enough, those who propose to view man as a machine are themselves caught in a dilemma. Machines, like men, cannot be reduced to their constituent parts. One does not recognize a radio by its physical and chemical components. Rather, a description of a radio indicates that it will transmit sound from one location to another. The fact that man may be characterized by some machine-like functions is not a valid basis on which to state that man is a machine. Machines are made by men and operate according to engineering principles basic to their design. On the other hand, the life process is a dynamic course which is continuous, creative, evolutionary, and uncertain. The patterning and organization of living systems are highly variable and constantly changing.

The functioning of organs and cells does not make them human beings. Respiratory systems, circulatory systems, neurological systems—individually or in the aggregate—no matter how thoroughly described, do not identify living systems.

The sentience of man cannot be reduced to systems, organs, and cells. Man's humanness is not the product of a machine. The wholeness of life cannot be identified in the laws of physics and biology. Moreover, "to represent living men as insentient is empirically false, but to regard them as thoughtful automata is logical nonsense."[21]

Neither can one view man's mind as a thing apart from the reality of his physicophysiological being and propose that this is man. Nor does one cross this bridge by identifying "mind" as an expression of neurological functioning. "The brain alone is not responsible for mind, even though it is a necessary organ for its manifestation. Indeed an isolated brain is a piece of biological nonsense."[22] Human beings are characterized by mass, structure, function, and feelings. They are not disembodied entities, nor are they mechanical aggregates. They are identifiable in their totality. They behave as a totality.

An energy field underwrites the unity of man and provides the conceptual boundaries which identify his oneness. Structure and function of living systems are field phenomena and reflect the dynamic nature of the life process. A field transcends its component parts. It possesses its own integrity. It acts as a whole. The human field is a starting point in envisioning the unity of man. *Human beings are more than and different from the sum of their parts.*

Human beings are identifiably people. No one mistakes a pancreas or a digestive system for a man. The distinctive properties that identify man emerge out of the study of man. One can describe the performance of an automobile without understanding its combustion system. So, too, can one describe the functioning of man without full knowledge of his particulate composition. This is not to deny the contribution of knowledge about man's particulate composition in furthering understanding of the nature of man. But man is visible only as his particulars disappear from view. The characteristics of man are those that identify his wholeness, his unity.

This unit is concerned with identifying and discussing some fundamental attributes of man. These attributes constitute a set of basic assumptions on which nursing science builds. The first of these assumptions (discussed in this chapter) may be stated thus:

Man is a unified whole possessing his own integrity and manifesting characteristics that are more than and different from the sum of his parts.

FOOTNOTES

1. deBroglie, Louis, *New Perspectives in Physics*, New York: Basic Books, Inc., Publishers, 1962, p. 68.

2. Mumford, Lewis, *The Transformations of Man*, New York: Harper & Brothers, 1956, p. 243.

3. Baranski, Leo J., *Scientific Basis for World Civilization*, Boston: The Christopher Publishing House, 1960.

4. Bergman, Peter G., *The Riddle of Gravitation*, New York: Charles Scribner's Sons, 1968.

5. deChardin, Teilhard, *The Phenomenon of Man*, New York: Harper and Row, 1961.

6. Dubos, René, *Man Adapting*, New Haven: Yale University Press, 1965.

7. duNoüy, Lecomte, *Human Destiny*, New York: Longmans, Green and Company, 1947.

8. Herrick, C. Judson, *The Evolution of Human Nature*, Austin, Texas: The University of Texas Press, 1956.

9. Koestler, Arthur, *The Ghost in the Machine*, New York: The Macmillan Company, 1968.

10. Polanyi, Michael, *Personal Knowledge*, Chicago, Ill.: The University of Chicago Press, 1958.

11. Virchow, R., "Atome und Individuen," *Vier Reden über Leben und Kranksein*, Berlin: 1862. (Translated by L. J. Rather as: "Atoms and Individuals," *Disease, Life, and Man*, Selected Essays by Rudolph Virchow, Stanford: Stanford University Press, 1958, pp. 120-141.)

12. Miller, James G., "Living Systems: Basic Concepts," *Behavioral Science*, Vol. 10, No. 3, July 1965, p. 213.

13. Miller, James G., "Living Systems: Cross-Level Hypotheses," *Behavioral Science*, Vol. 10, No. 4, October 1965, p. 407.

14. Miller, James G., "Living Systems: Basic Concepts," *Behavioral Science*, Vol. 10, No. 3, July 1965, p. 217.

15. Purcell, Edward, "Parts and Wholes in Physics," *Modern Systems Research for the Behavioral Scientist*, Chicago: Aldine Publishing Company, Inc., 1968, p. 43.

16. *Ibid.*, p. 44.

17. Bennett, J. G., *The Dramatic Universe*, London: Hodder and Stoughton. *The Foundations of Natural Philosophy*, Vol. I, 1956. *The Foundations of Moral Philosophy*, Vol. II, 1961. *Man and His Nature*, Vol. III, 1966. *History*, Vol. IV, 1966.

18. Bennett, J. G., *The Foundations of Natural Philosophy*, London: Hodder and Stoughton, 1956, p. 36.

19. As quoted in duNoüy, Lecomte, *Human Destiny*, New York: Longman, Green and Company, 1947, p. 19.

20. duNoüy, *op cit.*, pp. 17-18.

21. Polanyi, *op. cit.*, p. 339.

22. Huxley, Sir Julian, "Introduction" to deChardin, Teilhard, *The Phenomenon of Man*, New York: Harper and Row, 1961, p. 17.

CHAPTER 7

MAN: AN OPEN SYSTEM

"All things by immortal power
Near or far
Hiddenly
To each other linked are,
That thou canst not stir a flower
Without troubling of a star."

—Francis Thompson
The Mistress of Vision

People are inseparable from the natural world. As Henry Margenau has noted: "The universe does not flow around man. It flows through him."[1] The capacity of man and his surroundings to engage in a continuous interaction process rests on the fact that both are demonstrably open systems.

So thoroughly accepted is man's ongoing interaction with his environment that to emphasize that he is an open system may appear redundant. Despite its apparent obviousness, however, its implications for understanding man are by no means fully fathomed.

An open system is characterized by constant interchange of materials and energy with environment.[2] The growing field of human ecology rests firmly on the premise that man and nature are open systems. The term "ecosystem" has come into use "to mean the interaction system comprising living things and their environment."[3]

That environmental factors play an important role in man's becoming has had numerous proponents over past decades. Man's capacity to adapt to a wide range of environmental stresses has received considerable attention and has been proposed to be a significant factor in his survival. Homeostatic mechanisms have been described and adaptive responses to a range of selected variables have undergone scrutiny. General systems theorists propose models directed toward more effective quantification of data. Systems, sets, subsets have been incorporated into a vocabulary that permeates many segments of the scientific community. Ambiguous terminology is in process of further clarification.

But adaption and steady state, as traditionally construed, fail to explain the observable phenomenon of man's development. "Whereas adaptation blindly tries to attain an equilibrium which will bring about its end, evolution can only continue through unstable systems or organisms."[4]

The extent to which a concept of interaction that incorporates the notion of man and environment in dynamic interplay in which each is continually affecting and being affected by the other has been slow to permeate man's thinking. Claims to growing control over the environment abound. Natural laws are contravened. Myopic vision, expediency, and a sense of power over the forces of nature set in motion unforeseen changes of far-reaching import. In reality, though man may consciously rearrange and influence his environment, the environment is an ever-present and continuously active participant in the process of change. Moreover man's conscious efforts to determine and direct change have the further dimension of human and natural forces that are neither deliberate nor recognized.

Rachel Carson's *The Silent Spring* is a plea for seeing the long-range consequences of interfering with ecological relationships. Tuberculosis rates had already decreased markedly before the discovery of the tubercle bacillus and long before methods of prevention and cure had been proposed.[5] An air-conditioned room is scarcely reason for proclaiming control over prevailing atmospheric temperatures. The introduction of birth control "pills" to counteract the much-discussed population explosion may have outcomes quite different from those anticipated by the proponents of these drugs.

Though single causation has given way to a concept of multiple variables associated with human development and disease states, this too falls short of recognizing that man interacts as an integrated whole with the totality of the environment. Isolated variables indicative of subsystem and microscopic functioning are related to selected environmental factors. That a high correlation may be found between such components cannot be taken as a guarantee that changing a given environmental factor (s) will produce a particular effect. Change begets change, and change in any part creates change in the whole. Outcomes for the individual and society, when predictions are based on data that do not take into account the unity of man and his environment, may vary widely from anticipated results. The old truism that "the treatment was successful but the patient died" has its roots in reality.

Questions concerning man's place in nature reach back into antiquity. With the rise of modern science, evidence that man did not develop according to accepted physical laws became more explicit. Evolutionary theory furthered the recognition that living things developed in the direction of greater complexity in contrast to a physical world that was perceived to be moving toward homogeneity. The vital spirit, so dominant in the eighteenth century, became increasingly unsatisfactory as an explanation of human behavior.

The expansion of conventional physics to include the study of open systems as well as closed systems initiated the search for more fundamental unifying principles that were to have relevance for the biological as well as the physical world.

Contradictions between laws governing living and nonliving systems had long been recognized. Whereas naturally occurring processes in the physical world were observed to move in the direction of increasing disorder, living systems were characterized by increasing order. The second law of thermodynamics, useful in predicting the physical world, was inconsistent with the ways in which living systems behaved. Generally expressed, the second law states that "all naturally occurring processes tend to occur with change in entropy, and the change is always in the direction of an increase in entropy."[6] An increase in entropy posited a trend toward degradation to homogeneity of organization in contrast to a trend towards heterogeneity and complexity.

Failure of physical laws to explain the evolution of life led Ludwig von Bertalanffy[7] to explore a possible explanation for this contradiction. General systems theory[8] was introduced and the term negentropy was brought into use to signify increasing order, complexity, and heterogeneity. Living systems were said to be characterized by negentropy. C. Judson Herrick carried this thinking even further when he commented: "It may well be that the reversal of entropy is true for the cosmos as a whole and that the process of degradation that we call entropy is merely a local and transient episode in a vast domain of creative process that is continuously enlarging and progressively differentiating. In fact this possibility may be regarded as a probability, because there are no strictly closed systems in nature."[9]

Further limitations on the application of physical laws to living systems have been noted by Karl Trincher. Pointing out that the working processes of living matter contravene the second law of thermodynamics, Trincher[10] stated that cybernetics can imitate only those processes which follow the second law of thermodynamics.

Rapoport[11] endeavors to deal with this problem by stating that "no living system is a closed system and so the second law does not apply to it." He then goes on to demonstrate "how quasi-purposeful behavior can be manifested by an open physical system which is not necessarily 'alive' " and states that "non-living systems acquire *some* (Rapoport's italics) of the properties of living ones by virtue of being open." Such an approach would seem to emphasize the inadequacy of a mechanistic analogy to man rather than to strengthen it. Whether one speaks of machine-like characteristics in man or of man-like characteristics in machines, in neither instance is the integrity of the whole recognized.

Up to this point the identification of man's environment has been left in a rather nebulous state. Is environment to be conceived as that which is observably proximate to a given individual, or is it to be stretched beyond the limits of the known universe, or is it to be deemed to have its borders somewhere in between? Is it to be defined according to its constituent parts, either individually or collectively, or is it to be considered as a unified whole?

Hall and Fagen[12] have defined environment as follows: "For a given system, the environment is the set of all objects a change in whose attributes affects the system, and also those objects whose attributes are changed by the behavior of the system." This definition raises an immediate question. In a universe of open systems, how does one determine that a given set of objects is affecting and being affected by the system whereas other objects or sets of objects are not?

It is well known that man is subject to a range of influences that need not be physically at hand for their impact to be highly significant. In these days of rapid transit, family members may be long distances from one another. One would scarcely deny that the young child away at camp for the first time is nonetheless an influencing factor for his parents during his absence, and vice versa. Atomic bomb explosions have released radioactive fallout that may affect persons many miles beyond the original source of the explosion. More distant yet, the rays of the sun permeate our being. Who has not at some time said, "The sun is shining. How good I feel." Space research has revealed cosmic phenomena that not only add to the accuracy of weather prediction but are noted to be associated with man's health and well-being. Physicists identify smaller and smaller particles traveling at extraordinary speeds and continuously penetrating the energy field that is man.

Everyday life is replete with experiences that illustrate the validity of a concept of man affecting and being affected by the world about him. Concomitantly, the configuration of events occurring at any given point in time may include multiple variables of which man is unaware or which he may dismiss as of little or no consequence.

It is the *configuration* of events external to man that is a central factor in determining a definition of environment. A concept of patterning incorporates within it recognition that it is the totality of the constituents that compose the pattern. "Patterning" is a unifying concept. (See Chapter 9.) The unity of man has its counterpart in the unity of the environment. The environment possesses its own wholeness. Man-environment transactions are characterized by continuous repatterning of both man and environment.

Mushrooming scientific knowledge is rapidly adding a multiplicity of influences recognized to have their correlates with human development. It is no longer possible to conceive of man's environment as narrowed even to so sizable a unit as would be encompassed by the atmospheric boundaries of Earth. Man and his environment are coextensive with the universe. In view of man's miniscule knowledge about the universe, such a proposal may seem to belong more properly within the purview of literature and philosophy than of science. Furthermore, this statement implies a finite universe (a subject of much unresolved debate). It is not an easy matter to envision a universe of interacting wholes. Particularly is this true when one compares the known dimensions of man with the vastness of the universe and endeavors to relate the two. Nonetheless, in a universe in which there are no strictly closed systems, one cannot evade postulating man's environment as the patterned wholeness of all that is external to man. For individual man, environment is the patterned wholeness of all that is external to a given individual.

The constant interchange of matter and energy between man and environment is at the basis of man's becoming. It is this interchange that portends the creativity of life. It is in the mutual changing and being changed that evolution proceeds.

The second assumption on which nursing science builds may be stated thus:

Man and environment are continuously exchanging matter and energy with one another.

FOOTNOTES

1. Margenau, Henry, Paper presented at the Foundation for Integrative Education Lecture Series, February 23, 1965.

2. Bertalanffy, Ludwig von, "The Theory of Open Systems in Physics and Biology," *Science,* 111:23-25, January 13, 1950.

3. Evans, Francis C., "Ecosystems as the Basic Unit in Ecology," in E. V. Kormandy (Edit.) , *Readings in Ecology,* Englewood Cliffs, N. J.: Prentice-Hall, 1965, p. 166.

4 duNoüy, Lecomte, *Human Destiny,* New York: Longman, Green and Company, 1947, p. 90.

5. Dubos, René, *Man Adapting,* New Haven: Yale University Press, 1965, p. 166.

6. Baranski, Leo J., *Scientific Basis for World Civilization,* Boston: The Christopher Publishing House, 1960, p. 140.

7. Bertalanffy, *op. cit.,* p. 25.

8. Bertalanffy, Ludwig von, "General Systems Theory," *MAIN CURRENTS in Modern Thought,* Vol. 11, No. 4, March 1955, pp. 75-83.

9. Herrick, C. Judson, *The Evolution of Human Nature,* New York: Harper Torchbooks, 1961, p. 51.

10. Trincher, Karl S., *Biology and Information: Elements of Biological Thermodynamics* (authorized translation from the Russian by Edwin S. Spiegelthal) , New York: Consultants Bureau Enterprises, Inc., 1965.

11. Rapoport, Anatol, "Foreword," *Modern Systems Research for the Behavioral Scientist,* Chicago: Aldine Publishing Company, 1968, p. xviii.

12. Hall, R. D. and Fagen, R. E., "Definitions of a System," *General Systems Yearbook,* 1956.

CHAPTER **8**

THE UNIDIRECTIONALITY
OF LIFE

". . . the universe in its entirety must be regarded
as one gigantic process of becoming, of attaining new
levels of existence and organization which can properly be called a genesis or an evolution."
—Sir Julian Huxley

The evolutionary story of man's emergence covers many mil-
lennia. A continuous and continuing metamorphosis, demonstrably
innovative in character, marks both man and his environment.
Heterogeneity, diversification, and growing complexity are observable attributes of man's unfolding. The theory of progressive
evolution finds expression in man's sequential development. The
life process is a becoming. The evolution of life exhibits an invari-
ant one-way trend.

That living things contradict the second law of thermodynamics has already been noted in the previous chapter. The possibility
—nay, probability—that negentropy is a universal phenomenon is
emerging. Documentation of evolutionary events reveals the suc-
cessive nature of man's becoming and testifies to the inseparability
of environmental evolution in the process of change.

The process of change takes place in space along the time axis.
The concepts of past, present, and future denote time progression.
A perception of time passing is an integral part of man's everyday
life. "Time's Arrow" connotes that nothing will ever be the same
again. The notion of unidirectionality is reflected in Alfred Lord
Tennyson's words: "I am the heir of all the ages, in the foremost
files of time." The concept of evolution presupposes that time is
unidirectional. "The most conspicuous signs of the unidirectionality

of time can be traced to our participation in the general evolution of the universe."[1] The story of man's becoming is written in the constant transformation of energy that persists throughout the universe and finds expression in life's capacity to complexify.

A concept of universal becoming is not without its opponents. A static interpretation of space-time can be found both in the scientific literature and in the time machines of science fiction. Einstein[2] as late as 1949 was considering the possibility that the irreversibility of time was in reality a special case of Reichenbach's "world of the middle dimensions," not true on the cosmic scale and microphysical level. A becomingless view of space-time is expressed in Adolph Grünbaum's statement that "coming into being is only coming into awareness,"[3] a notion that persists in some psychological contexts today.

The relativistic fusion of space with time furthered a tendency to regard time as being essentially the same as space and to reinforce widely held static views of the physical world. At the same time, proposals to speak of "the dimension of time plus the three dimensions of space" reflected a view that time and space were not equivalent. Čapek has proposed that "the relativistic union of space with time is far more appropriately characterized as a *dynamization of space* rather than a spacialization of time."[4]

A need to examine "time" as a dimension in its own right and to explore the nature and meaning of its many aspects has led to a recent upsurge of literature on the subject.[5, 6, 7] Geological evolution is written in the rocks, and cosmic change is evidenced in the processes of star formation and development. The evolution of life has been traced in fossil records, in identification of growing complexity in life forms, and in discoveries of artifacts of man's emergence.

Louis Pasteur's "conclusive demonstration" in the 1860's that spontaneous generation of living organisms (abiogenesis) was not possible has contributed to a century of belief in the ancient history of all life forms. However, recent research[8] carried out at the University of Miami's Institute of Molecular Evolution suggests that the emergence of new life need not be limited to an earlier period when evolution had reached the point of producing the building blocks of life. Alongside the continuity of life through time is also evidence that new life may be originating spontaneously on Earth today. Such a proposal does not invalidate the historical evidence

some new development in man? Is the escalation of science and technology a reflection of escalation in the speed of human evolution?

Gene recombinations have been noted to be of greater significance than genetic mutations in the evolution of life.[10] With the advent of modern transportation, population mobility has grown by leaps and bounds. Communication media are making inroads on barriers established by cultural differences. Heretofore isolated societies are bypassing centuries of Western World development as they are introduced to the fruits of technology. The gene pools of the planet Earth are intermingling as never before and presage further evolutionary events.

Evidence of man's perceptual evolution is emerging as an increasing number of persons are being found to possess what Karagulla[11] calls "Higher Sense Perception." Man's traditional five senses (seeing, hearing, smelling, tasting, and touching), long deemed to be the means through which man learned about his world, are being supplemented by a new dimension. Investigations into the phenomena of creativity and extrasensory perception and a range of paranormal occurrences are opening up vast areas of conjecture about contemporary man's capacities for experiencing his world in ways perhaps less open to earlier peoples.

The future, like the past, is part of the evolutionary story of the universe. The irreversible and unidirectional nature of the life process is bound inextricably with the unfolding of the physical world. Increasing complexity and innovation mark the passing of time.

The third assumption on which nursing science builds may be stated thus:

The life process evolves irreversibly and unidirectionally along the space-time continuum.

FOOTNOTES

1. deBeauregard, Olivier Costa, "Relativity Theory: Arguments for a Philosophy of Being," *The Voices of Time* (edited by J. T. Fraser), New York: George Braziller, 1966, p. 431.

2. Čapek, Milič, "Time in Relativity Theory: Arguments for a Philosophy of Becoming," *The Voices of Time* (edited by J. T. Fraser), New York: George Braziller, 1966, p. 437.

3. Grünbaum, Adolph, *Philosophical Problems of Space and Time,* New York: Alfred Knopf, 1963, p. 329.

4. Čapek, Milič, *op. cit.,* p. 447.

5. Fischer, Roland (Editor), *Interdisciplinary Perspectives of Time,* New York: Alfred A. Knopf, 1963, p. 329.

6. Fraser, J. T. (Editor), *The Voices of Time,* New York: George Braziller, 1966.

7. Toulmin, S. and Goodfield, J., *The Discovery of Time,* New York: Harper Torchbooks, 1966.

8. Fox, S. W. and McCauley, R. J., "Could Life Originate Now?" *Natural History, August-September* 1968, pp. 26-30.

9. deChardin, Teilhard, *The Phenomenon of Man,* New York: Harper Torchbooks, 1961, p. 49.

10. Kalmus, Hans, "Organic Evolution and Time," *The Voices of Time* (edited by J. T. Fraser), New York: George Braziller, 1966, p. 352.

11. Karagulla, Shafica, *Breakthrough to Creativity,* California: DeVorss and Company, Inc., 1967.

CHAPTER **9**

LIFE'S PATTERN AND ORGANIZATION

". . . the world, harmoniously confused:
Where order in variety we see,
And where, though all things differ, all agree."

—Alexander Pope

That man is a highly complex organism is an accepted fact. The nature of this complexity and the characteristics of its governance have long troubled those who have tried to explain it. The search persists for fundamental theories that may shed light upon man's remarkable capacity to maintain himself while at the same time undergoing continuous change.

Pattern and organization have become basic concepts in contemporary efforts to achieve a better understanding of human growth and behavior. L. L. Whyte,[1] an English theorist, has postulated a universal creative-formative process which operates on a single principle and purposes to better explain the organization and patterning of life. General systems theorists study systems as entities instead of as aggregates of parts and seek to determine lawful processes in organizational growth. Pattern and organization are implicit in feed-back systems and in communication theory.

The existence of organization and patterning in living systems is an observable phenomenon. An energy field is the basic unit of living things. It is this field which imposes pattern and organization on the parts. It is pattern and organization that identifies man and and reflects his wholeness.

The presence of pattern and organization cannot be construed as a static phenomenon. The living system is an open system constantly exchanging matter and energy with the environment. The life process is dynamic—ever changing. It evolves toward growing complexity of organization—the unidirectional, negentropic qualities of life. The nature of life's pattern and organization is in constant process of evolution. Organization of the living system is maintained amidst kaleidoscopic alterations in patterning of the system. The irreversible nature of the life process prohibits repetition of pattern and foretells the innovative potentials of patterning.

Patterning of the living system subsumes within it both structure and function. These are dynamic processes. They are transcended by the life process and are inextricably merged in the wholeness of man's becoming. A static perception of structure, once in fashion, is in error. "What are called structures are slow processes of long duration, functions are quick processes of short duration."[2] In the wholeness of life, structure and function are united. As Whyte notes: "The concept of structure is valid only where the process of the whole can be neglected."[3] The life process possesses its own dynamic pattern and organization. The patterning that takes place over time is evolutionary in nature and encompasses the unity of life.

Pattern and organization are unifying concepts. They are observable properties of all there is. Without patterning there would be chaos. Without lawful development in nature there could be no meaningful predictions. The laws of probability reflect an orderly universe. The " 'formative process' is an intrinsic property of everything in the natural cosmos that is known to man."[4]

Further evidence of nature's lawfulness has come about through biorhythm research, expanded recognition of the cyclical nature of physical phenomena, and significant findings pointing up interrelationships between the two. The persistence of rhythmic relationships are noted in findings by marine biologists that oysters, moved inland from their native locations, will open and close while feeding according to the tide phases of the waters whence they came. Dubos speculates: "The high tides of the oceans may have their counterpart in the high tides of our blood stream."[5] A range of atmospheric phenomena have been found to be associated with various behavioral manifestations.[6, 7] The cycles of day and night have many predictable correlates in biochemical fluctuations.[8, 9]

Rhythmicity is a well documented concomitant of life and its environment. The unidirectionality of life proceeds rhythmically along a spiral. As each new curve of the spiral appears, cyclical continuity is revealed. What seems to be repetition is, in reality, only similarity. Events do not repeat themselves. Life's becoming is a continuous expression of negentropic change growing out of man-environment interaction. Becoming is an identifiably orderly process.

Patterning is a dynamic process. The continuous change that marks man and his environment is expressed in the continuing emergence of new patterns in man and environment. The order of the universe is maintained amidst constant change. So too does the patterning that identifies man undergo continuous revision and innovation. Man's capacity to maintain himself while undergoing continuous change is a remarkable characteristic. This capacity is commonly referred to as man's self-regulating ability.

Efforts to identify self-regulatory mechanisms operating in man have revealed a range of physiological factors noted to play significant roles in the maintenance of physiological functioning. In the 1930's W. B. Cannon[10] introduced the principle of homeostasis to indicate a relatively steady state of internal operation in the living system. More recently, findings growing out of the study of physiological cycles have pointed up critical inadequacies and inconsistencies in the concept of homeostasis.[11] The term homeokinesis has been introduced in an effort to more clearly portray the dynamic nature of biological functioning.

Feed-back mechanisms are proposed to be analogous to the self-regulatory process in man. However, these mechanisms provide only a model for certain machine-like operations taking place in man and have critical limitations when applied to living systems. Ashby[12] has pointed out: "Such complex systems cannot be treated as an interlaced set of more or less independent feedback circuits, but only as a whole" and goes on to state: "For understanding the general principles of dynamic systems, therefore, the concept of feedback is inadequate in itself."

Ability to comprehend man as an organized whole possessing his own identity, and as more than and different from the sum of his parts, should take on further clarity as the concept of patterning is understood. In conceptualizing a complex whole, the Black Box model may prove helpful. The Black Box theory assumes an encased whole within which the internal mechanisms are not open to examination. This theory provides that the system under study be equipped with input-output terminals and directs attention to the properties of the system and not to its contents.

Suppose one visualizes the energy field of man as a whole encased in a permeable boundary contiguous with the permeable boundary of the environment. Input-output is continuous between the two, with concomitant and constant alterations in the patterning of both man and environment. At the same time that the contents of an energy field are in continuous flux, the identity of the field as a whole is maintained. In the input-output process, the changing contents affect the field, and the field imposes pattern and organization upon the contents. It is pattern and organization which give meaning to the field. Furthermore, "all particulars become meaningless if we lose sight of the pattern which they jointly constitute."[13] The properties of the living system have their meaning in the patterning and organization of the system and not in the particulars of the system.

The patterning of life is evolutionary in nature. The creative-formative process is integral to man and his environment and basic to understanding the man-environment relationship. It is the continuous repatterning of man and environment along life's axis that characterizes the dynamic nature of the universe. Self-regulation is directed toward achieving increasing complexity of organization—*not* toward achieving equilibrium and stability.

The capacity of life to transcend itself is contrary to theories that propose the goals of life are adaptive in nature. Maslow has commented: "Homeostasis, equilibrium, adaptation, self-preservation, defense, and adjustment are merely negative concepts and must be supplemented by positive concepts.[14] Kurt Goldstein[15] strongly disagreed with motivational theory which assumed that reduction of tension, and thus reestablishment of equilibrium, was the basic motive. Frankl[16] supports the view that self-regulation is not for the purpose of reducing tensions but, on the contrary, for maintaining tensions. Freud's pleasure principle does not stand up under the evidence of life's negentropic evolution. The regulatory process in man is directed toward diversity. By virtue of life's probabilistic goal seeking, it is characterized by constraints and at the same time is an expression of creative-formative process. The orderliness of nature is of itself a constraint against randomness and chaos. Self-regulation is a dynamic quality directed toward orderly innovation.

Self-regulation is directed toward fulfilling the potentialities of life. That facets of this process go on even though an individual may not be consciously deliberating upon them is well known. At the same time, man has the capacity to knowingly rearrange his environment and to exercise choices in fulfilling his potentialities. Self-regulating mechanisms of the physiological organism are identified with maintaining multiple functions in the living system. Concomitantly, a range of physiological functions are demonstrably subject to conscious control. Self-regulation is an expression of wholeness. It cannot be explained by subsystem functioning.

The identification of wholeness rests in the patterning and organization of that which is to be identified. Recognition of patterns as a means of distinguishing individuals is an everyday occurrence. Not only are individuals identified by the wholeness of pattern but perception of the nature of the pattern is reflected in such verbalizations as "Mary Smith is sad." Mary Smith's sadness is an expression of wholeness, not of Mary Smith's particulate composition. If Mary Smith's observer is asked to explain why he thinks Mary Smith is sad, he may respond with such a broad generality as "I can tell by looking at her," thus expressing the unity of his perception.

Pattern and organization are fundamental attributes of all there is. They give unity to diversity and reflect a dynamic and creative universe.

The fourth assumption on which nursing science builds may be stated thus:

Pattern and organization identify man and reflect his innovative wholeness.

FOOTNOTES

1. Whyte, Lancelot Law, *The Next Development in Man,* New York: The New American Library, 1950.

2. Bertalanffy, Ludwig von, *Problems of Life,* New York: John Wiley and Sons, Inc., 1952, p. 134.

3. Whyte, L. L., *op. cit.,* p. 19.

4. Herrick, C. J., *The Evolution of Human Nature,* New York: Harper and Brothers, 1956, p. 60.

5. Dubos, René, *Man Adapting,* New Haven: Yale University Press, 1965, p. 49.

6. Sollberger, A., *Biological Rhythm Research,* New York: Elsevier Publishing Company, 1965.

7. Wolf, William (Editor), *Rhythmic Functions in the Living System* (Annals of the New York Academy of Sciences, Vol. 98, Art. 4), New York: New York Academy of Sciences, October 30, 1962.

8. Sollberger, A., *loc. cit.*

9. Wolf, William, *loc. cit.*

10. Cannon, W. B., *The Wisdom of the Body,* second edition, New York: Norton Publishing Company, 1939.

11. Shaefer, Karl E. (Editor), *Man's Dependence on the Earthly Atmosphere,* New York: The Macmillan Company, 1962, p. viii.

12. Ashby, W. Ross, *Cybernetics,* New York: John Wiley and Sons, Inc., 1963, p. 54.

13. Polanyi, Michael, *Personal Knowledge,* Chicago: The University of Chicago Press, 1958, p. 57.

14. Maslow, A. H., *Motivation and Personality,* New York: Harper and Row, 1954, p. 367.

15. Goldstein, Kurt, *The Organism,* New York: American Book Company, 1939.

16. Frankl, Viktor E., *Psychotherapy and Existentialism,* New York: Simon and Schuster, 1968.

CHAPTER **10**

MAN: A SENTIENT, THINKING BEING

"Man, unlike any other thing organic or inorganic in the universe, grows beyond his work, walks up the stairs of his concepts, emerges ahead of his accomplishments."

—John Ernst Steinbeck

The material presented in the preceding four chapters has relevance for all living systems, not just man. The expressions of wholeness, interaction, unidirectionality, and pattern reveal themselves in a wide range of living creatures identifiably different from one another. The commonalities of life are transcended in the differentiation of orders, classes, and species. The organization of life encompasses the simplest organism to the most complex in an evolutionary hierarchy of development ordered along the phylogenetic scale. At the top of this scale man stands triumphant, reveling in his uniqueness and in his achievements.

What is there about man that he is not only different from other living forms but that he is in the forefront of evolutionary complexity? Is he really as unique as he likes to think himself? Surely, as man's knowledge of the universe expands, man's place within it shrinks before his growing awareness of the immensity of the unknown. And herein lies the uniqueness of man. Of the earth's life forms, only man perceives and ponders the vastness of the cosmos. What other living creature is aware of his evolutionary past? Who but man envisions a future? Abstraction and imagery, language and thought, sensation and emotion are fundamental attributes of man's humanness.

Man's awareness of himself and his world is rooted in cognizance of his own mortality. Prehistory has left its artifacts of man's concern with death. Religious rituals, art forms, and speculative philosophy attest to man's continuing search through time for the meaning of life and death. The value of man can be found in the human sacrifices which at one time were deemed the acme for propitiation of the gods. Mandates against the killing of men thread far back into man's history. Promises of a hereafter hedge the fears associated with man's passing.

Contemporary man endeavors to postpone death as long as possible. Organ transplants, the human deep-freeze, and perpetuation of vital signs past any hope of reversing the dying process are indicative of man's efforts to hold back the "grim reaper." Only recently has recognition of the dignity of death and of the rights of the dying begun to emerge in U.S. culture, though such concern is a significant facet of certain other cultures.

Man's concern for perpetuation of life is filled with paradoxes. Notwithstanding efforts throughout the United States to ban the death penalty, legal death is still a reality. Wars continue. The adolescent's comment that he "doesn't want to become a statistic" grew out of the rising death toll on the nation's highways. Despite man's urge to live, he nonetheless dares exploration of mountain tops and ocean depths; challenges the multiple unknowns of outer space; and dies, gloriously or ingloriously as the case may be, for an idea.

The continuity of life is maintained through reproduction. The cycle of life and death is a rhythmic correlate of the continuity of life. Individual death is a condition of living. The meaning of death is a personal one. Man's awareness of his mortality is a strictly human condition. How man meets death, the meaning he attaches to it, and the beliefs he holds relative to after death reveal his gropings for cosmic understanding.

Man is a sentient being. Though man is not alone in possessing the capacity to feel, the depth and scope of his feelings extend far beyond those of other animals. Susan Langer[1] uses feeling "to designate *anything that may be felt*" (Langer's italics). Within this context then, sensation and emotion are felt responses to the environment. Feeling is used in its broadest sense.

Man experiences feelings as a unified being. Feelings are an expression of wholeness. Love cannot be described as the product of some disembodied entity nor can the ache of a tooth be truly explained by the presence of an exposed nerve. Feelings are field functions and as such encompass the totality of the individual. The inadequacies of psychology or biology to explain feelings on the basis of either mind or matter are multiple. The relatively new field of psychobiology reflects some of these difficulties. Pain thresholds vary widely from one individual to another and neither psychology nor biology has found an answer. Biochemical correlates of fear, anger, courage, relaxation scarcely explain the imagery, abstraction, and thought (unique to man) that give these feelings human meaning. L.S.D. visions are said to expand man's consciousness. But consciousness itself is a vague and ambiguous term.

Historically the study of feelings has been predominantly allocated to the realm of psychology. Today's "behavioral sciences," in their efforts to become more "scientific," are oriented toward factual description and, more often than not, relegate feelings and subjective experience to the metaphysical.[2] Only overt behavior is deemed valid for study and inward experience is overlooked, if not denied, by the behaviorists. Mechanistic analogies and mathematical formulas further serve to deny human sentience as a proper area for investigation. One might propose that a mechanistic explanation of behavior with its application to the real world may be far more dehumanizing than today's onrush of automation and job displacements. Carl Rogers' comment: "The warm, subjective encounter of two persons is more effective in facilitating change than is the most precise set of techniques growing out of learning theory or operant conditioning"[3] needs careful thought. It seems unlikely, for example, that the "battered child syndrome" could yield to an extrapolation of overt facts and a set of stimulus-response activities. There are those, of course, who deem man's feelings proper subjects for study. The exploration of man's need to work through grief is an illustration of such interest.

Man feels. His sentience finds expression in joy and sorrow, ecstasy and depression, affection, zeal. He feels the colors of a sunset, the strains of a Bach, the sweep of a horizon. He mourns with Milton the death of Lycidus and laughs with glee at the antics of Barnum and Bailey's clowns. He feels the touch of velvet and the aroma of fresh coffee, the prick of a pin and the chill of isolation.

Feelings are subjective. Language does not suffice to transmit their personal nature. But language does provide a singularly human means for transmitting thought, for preserving the past, and for anticipating the future. Language is more than sounds denoting objects. It is the means whereby man communicates ideas and abstractions. Language is a tool of logic and reason, with mathematics the most abstract language of all.

Man seeks to organize the world of his experience and to make sense of it. The web of understanding that transcends the accumulation of facts and events arises out of man's capacity for rational thought. The emergence of modern science brought with it a stereotype of cold appraisal and carefully organized objectivity in which value judgments are denied. So masterful have been the methods of science in revealing new knowledge and in providing man with a wealth of technological wonders that both honor and dollars attend its workers and its works. As the industrial era dimmed in the bright light of atomic discoveries and cybernetics, men grew fearful that machines and robots would soon replace them. Scientific humanitarianism (or humanitarian scientism if the reader prefers) crept upon the scene.

Strange as it may seem to those who proclaim their dedication to a clearly delineated formalization of scientific method, it is feelings that provide the basic motivation for inquiry no matter how inflexible may be the rules that govern exploration. The "science for science's sake" dictum is underwritten by a drive for knowing, for experiencing the joy of discovery. Efforts to alleviate the human predicament through scientific study and its application are rooted in social awareness. As remarkable as are the science and technology that daily cross new frontiers, they are not nearly so remarkable as the expansion of man's thought and emotions which make the crossings possible.

Frankl[4, 5] has proposed that man's basic need is to find meaning in life—and in death. Multiple cosmologies are advanced to explain man's place in the universe. Youth cries out for relevance and seeks confrontation for relief of frustration in the "will-to-meaning". Philosophy and religion, the arts and sciences, each in its own way, look upon man's humanness and reflect his quandary. But out of the human dilemma there does arise a personal meaning. Logic and reason alone do not suffice to give this meaning. Rather, man's capacity for imagery and abstraction, language and thought, sensation and emotion combine to express man's humanness and to open up broad avenues to understanding. Perhaps

Pythagoras was expressing this when he said: "There is geometry in the humming of the strings. There is music in the spacing of the spheres."

Feelings as well as rational thought are positive integrating forces. The world of man's experience is ordered in the beauty of a mountain topped with snow, in the sound of music, in the grief of personal loss, in the pain of physical hurt. Concomitantly, feelings alone cannot provide the means whereby man is enabled to grope toward understanding. Language and thought are indispensable to man's growing awareness of himself and his world. Without logic and reason, man's efforts to better himself and the human condition would surely fall awry. Unreasoning and unreasonable men destroy the very foundations of man's search for meaning.

A growing capacity to perceive relationships between events and to hypothesize new relationships marks man's evolution through time. Concept formation—the ordering of thought—is basic to organized action.

Sentience and thought are integral to the vital process itself. The patterning of the human field is more than an assembling and reassembling of parts directed toward automatic self-regulatory acts. Man knowingly makes choices. Through awareness of himself and his environment, he is an active participant in determining the patterning of his field and in reorganizing the environment in accord with his desires. His choices are not necessarily wise ones. Some choices may even be detrimental to his well-being. Failure to make a choice is of itself a decision that is incorporated into the man-environment interaction process.

Man's potential for conscious involvement in the self-regulatory process is little understood. Even less understood is the evolutionary creativity that is going on continuously and that is postulated to express itself in identifiable, growing complexity of organization and patterning in man and environment. There is a popularly held belief that man's scientific and technological know-how has outstripped his cultural development. Such a view denies man's wholeness and ignores the universality of unidirectional creative evolution. Moreover, there is blindness to the creative evolution that affects form and structure of man as well as the concomitant social and environmental milieu. Can homo sapiens expect to remain forever at the top of the phylogenetic scale? Arthur C. Clarke, more than a decade ago, in commenting on man's advent into outer space, wrote: "What is happening now is nothing less than the next stage in evolution, comparable to the time, perhaps a billion years ago, when life came out of the sea and conquered the land"[6]

The creativity of life is a continually evolving phenomenon. Evidence of this creativity finds further expression in the changing dimensions of man's sentience and thought. They are integral to the life process itself. In the process of interaction between man and environment, man's self-knowledge and knowledge of his world emerge.

Man's knowledge of his world has long been deemed to come through his five senses (taste, smell, sight, sound, and touch). In recent years scientific respectability has been granted to the study of extrasensory phenomena. The existence of paranormal occurences is well documented. There are persons whose knowledge of the world is augmented by information gained through other than the five senses. Probably this has been true of visionaries of centuries past as well as now. Today, however, it seems likely that a much larger number of people possess some powers of extrasensory perception and that this capacity can be enhanced through training, even though testable hypotheses to explain it are still in short supply.

Man's feelings and thoughts are not limited to the waking state. Numerous investigations into the electrical correlates of sleep have found them to be associated with dreaming. Efforts to interpret the meanings of dreams appear frequently in the psychoanalytic literature. Dreams are often noted to be associated with paranormal phenomena. They are also blamed on indigestion and overexcitement. The night terrors of young children are so common that parents are frequently advised to have little concern over their occurrence. Anxiety, irritability, and an increase in appetite have been reported to occur in persons deprived of dreaming.[7] Dreams provide a further means whereby integration and patterning of life occur.

Evolution in the sleep-wake cycle is becoming increasingly evident. Changes in the sleep-wake pattern are characteristic of growth and development from infancy through old age. Whereas young children generally sleep approximately two-thirds of the 24-hour period, the reverse is true for adults.[8] In the agrarian era, man's sleep-wake cycle tended to follow the setting and rising of the sun. With the advent of the industrial age, man's pattern of sleep-wake periods began to show an observable shift. Twentieth century man has been told he needed eight hours of sleep each night. Recent research findings have shortened this to seven hours as being most compatible with healthy functioning. Does man's apparently diminished need for sleep portend growing awareness in the waking state? Is extrasensory perception an evolutionary emergent integral to these changes?

Man's capacity for experiencing himself and his world identifies his humanness. Abstract thought couched in language enables him to grope toward cosmic understanding. The arts and sciences, philosophy and religion attest to man's evolutionary potential with transcendence of his present self.

The fifth assumption on which nursing science builds may be stated thus:

Man is characterized by the capacity for abstraction and imagery, language and thought, sensation and emotion.

FOOTNOTES

1. Langer, Susan, *Philosophical Sketches,* New York: The New American Library of World Literature, 1964, p. 16.
2. Langer, S., *op. cit.,* p. 13.
3. Rogers, Carl, "Two Divergent Trends," *Existential Psychology,* edited by Rollo May, New York: Random House, Inc., 1961, p. 93.
4. Frankl, Viktor, *Man's Search for Meaning,* New York: Washington Square Press, Inc., 1963.
5. Frankl, Viktor, *Psychotherapy and Existentialism,* New York: Simon and Schuster, 1968.
6. Clarke, Arthur C., *The Challenge of the Spaceship,* New York: Ballantine Books, 1961, p. 145.
7. Dement, W. C., The Effect of Dream Deprivation," *Science,* 131:1705-1707; 132:1420-1422, 1960.
8. Kleitman, Nathaniel, *Sleep and Wakefulness,* Chicago: University of Chicago Press (Revised and Enlarged Edition), 1963.

RELATED READINGS

ALLPORT, GORDON W., *Becoming: Basic Considerations for a Psychology of Personality,* New Haven: Yale University Press, 1955.

ANDREWS, DONALD HATCH, *The Symphony of Life,* Lee's Summit, Missouri: Unity Books, 1966.

ASHBY, W. ROSS, *Cybernetics,* New York: John Wiley & Sons, Inc., 1963.

BARANSKI, LEO J., *Scientific Basis for World Civilization: Unitary Field Theory,* Boston: The Christopher Publishing House, 1960.

BARRETT, WILLIAM, *Irrational Man,* New York: Doubleday and Co., Inc., 1962.

BASS, ROBERT, "Unity of Nature," *Human Biology,* XXIII:323-327, 1951.

BELLMAN, RICHARD, *Adaptive Control Processes*, Princeton, New Jersey: Princeton University Press, 1961.

BENNETT, J. G., *The Dramatic Universe: The Foundations of Natural Philosophy* (Vol. I) , London: Hodder & Stoughton, 1956.

———, *The Dramatic Universe: The Foundations of Moral Philosophy* (Vol. II) , London: Hodder & Stoughton, 1961.

———, *The Dramatic Universe: Man and His Nature* (Vol. III) , London: Hodder & Stoughton, 1966.

———, *The Dramatic Universe: History* (Vol. IV) , London: Hodder & Stoughton, 1968.

Berelson, B. and Steiner, G., *Human Behavior*, New York: Harcourt, Brace and World, Inc., 1964.

Berne, Eric, *Games People Play*, New York: Grove Press, Inc., 1964.

Bertalanffy, Ludwig von, "The Theory of Open Systems in Physics and Biology," *Science*, 111:23-25, January 13, 1950.

———, "General Systems Theory," *MAIN CURRENTS in Modern Thought*, Vol. 11, No. 4, March 1955.

———, *Robots, Men and Minds*, New York: George Braziller, 1967.

BONNER, JAMES, *The Molecular Biology of Development*, New York: Oxford University Press, 1965.

BORGESE, ELIZABETH MANN, *The Language Barrier: Beasts and Man*, New York: Holt, Rinehart and Winston, 1965.

BRONOWSKI, J., "The Clock Paradox," *Scientific American*, February 1963.

———, *Science and Human Values*, New York: Harper Torchbooks, 1965.

BROŽEK, JOSEF (Edit.) , *The Biology of Human Variation*, New York: New York Academy of Sciences, 1966.

BUBER, MARTIN, *I and Thou* (second edition) , New York: Charles Scribner's Sons, 1958.

BUCKLEY, WALTER (Edit.) , *Modern Systems Research for the Behavioral Scientist*, Chicago: Aldine Publishing Company, 1968.

BÜNNING, ERWIN, *The Physiological Clock*, New York: Academic Press, Inc., 1964.

CANDLAND, DOUGLAS (Edit.) , *Emotion: Bodily Change*, New York: D. Van Nostrand Company, Inc., 1962.

CANNON, W. B., *The Wisdom of the Body* (second edition) , New York: Norton Publishing Company, 1939.

CARRIGHAR, SALLY, *Wild Heritage*, Boston: Houghton Mifflin, 1965.

CLARKE, ARTHUR C., *The Challenge of the Spaceship*, New York: Ballantine Books, 1961.

DEBROGLIE, LOUIS, "The Philosophical Meaning and Practical Consequences of Cybernetics," *New Perspectives in Physics*, New York: Basic Books, 1962.

DECHARDIN, PIERRE TEILHARD, *The Phenomenon of Man*, New York: Harper and Row, 1961.

DOBZHANSKY, THEODOSIUS, *Heredity and the Nature of Man*, New York: Harcourt, Brace and World, 1964.

———, "Changing Man," *Science*, Vol. 155, No. 3761, January 27, 1967, pp. 409-414.

DUBOS, RENÉ, *Man Adapting*, New Haven: Yale University Press, 1965.

DUNOÜY, LECOMTE, *Human Destiny*, New York: Longmans, Green and Co., 1947.

EINSTEIN, ALBERT, *Relativity*, New York: Crown Publishing Co., Inc., 1961.

FEIFEL, HERMAN (Edit.) , *The Meaning of Death*, New York: McGraw-Hill Book Co., Inc., 1959. (Paperback edition, 1965.)

FISCHER, ROLAND (Edit.), *Interdisciplinary Perspectives of Time*, Annals of the New York Academy of Sciences, Vol. 138, Art. 2, New York: New York Academy of Sciences, February 6, 1967.

FOX, S. W. and MCCAULEY, R. J., "Could Life Originate Now?," *Natural History*, August-September 1968, pp. 26-30.

FRANKL, VIKTOR E., *Man's Search for Meaning*, New York: Washington Square Press, Inc., 1963.

———, *Psychotherapy and Existentialism*, New York: Simon and Schuster, 1968.

FRASER, J. T. (Edit.), *The Voices of Time*, New York: George Braziller, Inc., 1966.

FULTON, ROBERT (Edit.), *Death and Identity*, New York: John Wiley & Sons, Inc., 1965.

GANOW, GEORGE, "The Principle of Uncertainty," *Scientifie American*, January 1958.

GOLDSTEIN, KURT, *The Organism*, New York: American Book Co., 1939.

GRINKER, ROY R. (Edit.), *Toward a Unified Theory of Human Behavior*, New York: Basic Books, Inc., Publishers, 1967.

GRÜNBAUM, ADOLPH, *Philosophical Problems of Space and Time*, New York: Alfred A. Knopf, 1963.

HAIMOWITZ, M. L. and HAIMOWITZ, N. R. (Edit.), *Human Development*, New York: Thomas Y. Crowell Company, 1960.

HALL, EDWARD T., *The Hidden Dimension*, New York: Doubleday & Co., Inc., 1966.

HEBB, D. O., *The Organization of Behavior*, New York: John Wiley & Sons, Inc., 1949.

HEISENBERG, WERNER, *Physics and Philosophy*, New York: Harper and Brothers, 1958.

HEMPEL, CARL G., "General Systems Theory and the Unity of Science," *Human Biology*, XXIII:313-322, 1951.

HERRICK, C. JUDSON, *The Evolution of Human Nature*, Austin, Texas: University of Texas Press, 1956.

HOOK, SIDNEY, *The Quest for Being*, New York: Dell Publishing Co., A Delta Book, 1961.

JOUVET, MICHEL, "The States of Sleep," *Scientific American*, February 1967, pp. 62-72.

KARAGULLA, SHAFICA, *Breakthrough to Creativity*, California: DeVorss & Co., Inc., 1967.

KASTENBAUM, ROBERT (Edit.), *Psychobiology of Aging*, New York: Springer Publishing Co., Inc., 1965.

KILPATRICK, F. P., *Explorations in Transactional Psychology*, New York: New York University Press, 1961.

KING, DALY, *The States of Human Consciousness*, New York: University Books, 1963.

KLEITMAN, NATHANIEL, *Sleep and Wakefulness*, Chicago: The University of Chicago Press, 1965.

KOESTLER, ARTHUR, *The Act of Creation*, New York: The Macmillan Co., 1964.

———, *The Ghost in the Machine*, New York: The Macmillan Co., 1968.

KORMANDY, E. V. (Edit.), *Readings in Ecology*, Englewood Cliffs, New Jersey: Prentice-Hall, 1965.

KRECH, DAVID, *Individual in Society*, New York: McGraw-Hill Book Co., 1962.

LANDAUER, THOMAS K. (Edit.), *Readings in Physiological Psychology*, New York: McGraw-Hill Book Co., 1967.

LANGER, SUSAN, *Philosophical Sketches*, New York: The New American Library of World Literature, 1964.

——, *Mind: An Essay on Human Feeling, Volume I*. Baltimore: The Johns Hopkins Press, 1967.

LUCKEY, THOMAS D., *Germfree Life and Gnotobiology*, New York: Academic Press, 1963.

MANNION, ALAN, "Self-Regulation: A Unified Attack on the Problem," *MAIN CURRENTS in Modern Thought*, Vol. 16, No. 1, September 1959.

MARGENAU, HENRY, "Particle and Field Concepts in Biology," *Scientific Monthly*, 64:225-231, 1947.

——, "Fields in Physics and Biology," *MAIN CURRENTS in Modern Thought*, Vol. 15, No. 3, 1959.

MASLOW, A. H., *Motivation and Personality*, New York: Harper and Row, 1954.

—— (Edit.), *New Knowledge in Human Values*, New York: Harper & Brothers, 1959.

MAY, ROLLO (Edit.), *Existential Psychology*, New York: Random House, Inc., 1961.

MENNINGER, KARL, *The Vital Balance*, New York: Viking Press, 1963.

MILLER, JAMES G., "Living Systems: Basic Concepts," *Behavioral Science*, Vol. 10, No. 3, July 1965, pp. 193-237.

——, "Living Systems: Structure and Process," *Behavioral Science*, Vol. 10, No. 4, October 1965, pp. 337-379.

——, "Living Systems: Cross-Level Hypothesis," *Behavioral Science*, Vol. 10, No. 4, October 1965, pp. 380-411.

MORRIS, DESMOND, *The Naked Ape*, New York: McGraw-Hill Book Co., 1967.

MUMFORD, LEWIS, *The Transformations of Man*, New York: Harper & Brothers, 1956.

MURCHIE, GUY, *Music of the Spheres*, Boston: Houghton-Mifflin Company, 1961.

MURPHY, GARDNER, *Human Potentialities*, New York: Basic Books, Inc., 1958.

NETTLESHIP, ANDERSON, "The Entetechy of Time," *MAIN CURRENTS in Modern Thought*, Vol. 15, No. 3, January 1959.

NEUMANN, ERICH, *The Origins and History of Consciousness*, Vol. I. New York: Harper & Brothers, 1962.

POLANYI, MICHAEL, *Personal Knowledge*, Chicago, Illinois: The University of Chicago Press, 1958.

PORTMAN, ADOLF, *New Paths in Biology*, New York: Harper & Brothers, 1964.

REICHENBACH, HANS, *The Philosophy of Space and Time*, New York: Dover Publications, Inc., 1958.

REINBERG, ALAIN AND GHATA, JEAN, Biological Rhythms, New York: Walker and Co., 1964.

REISMAN, DAVID, *The Lonely Crowd*, Garden City, New York: Doubleday Anchor Books, 1950.

ROSSI, BRUNO, *Cosmic Rays*, New York: McGraw-Hill Book Co., 1964.

SELYE, HANS, *The Stress of Life*, New York: McGraw-Hill Book Co., 1956.

SHAEFFER, KARL E. (Edit.), *Man's Dependence on the Earthly Atmosphere*, New York: The Macmillan Co., 1962.

SINNOTT, EDMUND, *Cell and Psyche*, New York: Harper Torchbooks, 1961.

SOLLBERGER, A., *Biological Rhythm Research*, New York: Elsevier Publ. Co., 1965.

STEVENSON, IAN, *Twenty Cases Reminiscent of Reincarnation*, New York: American Society for Psychical Research, 1966.

SULLIVAN, WALTER, *We Are Not Alone*, New York: McGraw-Hill Book Co., 1964.

TAYLOR, C. W. and BARRON, F. (Edit.), *Scientific Creativity*, New York: John Wiley & Sons, Inc., 1963.

THOMPSON, D'ARCY W., *On Growth and Form*, Cambridge: Cambridge University Press, 1961.

TOULMIN, S. and GOODFIELD, J., *The Architecture of Matter*, New York: Harper Torchbooks, 1966.

——, *The Discovery of Time*, New York: Harper Torchbooks, 1966.

TRINCHER, KARL S., *Biology and Information: Elements of Biological Thermodynamics* (authorized translation from the Russian by Edwin S. Spiegelthal), New York: Consultants Bureau Enterprises, Inc., 1965.

U. S. Department of Health, Education, and Welfare, *Current Research on Sleep and Dreams*, Superintendent of Documents, U. S. Government Printing Office, Washington, D.C. 20402. (65¢)

WEINER, NORBERT, *The Human Use of Human Beings*, New York: Doubleday & Co., 1954.

WHITEHEAD, A. N., *Adventures of Ideas*, New York: The New American Library, 1960.

WHYTE, LANCELOT, *The Next Development in Man*, New York: Mentor Books, 1948.

—— (Edit.), *Aspects of Form*, Bloomington: Indiana University Press, Midland Book Edition, 1961.

WOLF, WILLIAM (Edit.), *Rhythmic Functions in the Living System*, Annals of the New York Academy of Sciences, Vol. 98, Art. 4, New York: New York Academy of Sciences, October 30, 1962.

WOLSTENHOLME, G. E. W. and MILLAR, E. C. P (Edit.), *Extrasensory Perception*, Boston: Little, Brown and Company, 1956.

ZIRKLE, R., "A Biophysical Symposium: The Particle Approach to Biology," *Scientific Monthly*, 64:213-216, 1947.

The Anatomy of Sleep, Nutley, New Jersey. Roche Laboratories, 1966.

NURSING'S CONCEPTUAL SYSTEM

UNIT III

"To venture causes anxiety. But not to venture is to lose oneself."

—Sören Kierkegaard

INTRODUCTION TO
UNIT III

Nursing exists to serve people. The extent to which nurses will be successful in contributing to the health and welfare of human beings is dependent on the nature and validity of the hard core of theoretical knowledge that underwrites nursing practice.

The science of nursing is not a summation of facts and principles drawn from other sources. Nursing's science is an emergent—a new product. The unifying principles and hypothetical generalizations basic to nursing seek to describe, explain, and predict about the phenomenon central to nursing's purpose—Man.

A body of scientific knowledge requires that there be clear, unequivocal concepts out of which theories can develop. Theories must be tested and retested against reality to determine their validity and reliability. Never will the results of testing have absolute certainty. The elaboration of any science is replete with eliminations and additions, revisions and alterations. Nonetheless, despite the probabilistic nature of scientific findings and the potential for error in all knowing, prediction remains a primary tool in determining meaningful intervention directed toward achieving human health and welfare. The level of confidence one can place in any prediction has substantive significance for people.

Description, explanation, and prediction are the predecessors of knowledgeable intervention. Nursing's theoretical system is built upon the basic assumptions discussed in Unit II. In the present unit, a conceptual model of the living system, man, is proposed. Unifying principles are identified and empirical support arising out of nursing research is discussed. Hopefully the ideas presented in Unit III will stimulate much critical thinking. There is grave need for basic research in nursing that will 1) further the formulation of nursing's system of concepts, 2) result in synthesis of knowledges for new concepts, and 3) be characterized by the creative development of testable hypotheses.

Nursing is committed to maintaining and promoting human health and to providing evaluative, therapeutic, and rehabilitative services to people. The elaboration of nursing's theoretical system is indispensable to fulfilling this commitment. Compassionate concern for human beings gives meaning to the effort. For those in nursing who join in exploring the unknown there awaits the joy of discovery.

CHAPTER 11

THE AIMS OF NURSING SCIENCE

"The central aims of science are . . . concerned with a search for understanding—a desire to make the course of nature not just predictable but intelligible."

—Stephen Toulmin

The science of nursing is an emergent—a new product. The inevitability of its development is written in nursing's long commitment to human health and welfare. With today's rapid and unprecedented changes, new urgency has been added to the critical need for a body of scientific knowledge specific to nursing. Only as the science of nursing takes on form and substance can the art of nursing achieve new dimensions of artistry. Knowledgeable nursing services are indispensable to public safety. Humanitarian values add a further imperative to the search for understanding man and his world.

The predictive principles needed to guide nursing practice emerge out of nursing's conceptual system. Science seeks to make intelligible the world of man's experiences. Nursing science seeks to make intelligible knowledge about man and his world that has special significance for nursing. The phenomenon central to nursing's conceptual system is the life process in man. A conceptual model of the life process in man (See Chapter 12) provides the base from which relevant theories may be derived and tested.

Science is concerned with meanings rather than with facts. A conceptual frame of reference is an indispensable prerequisite to the ordering of knowledges and to the formulation of meaningful propositions. An organized system of concepts further provides a repository for experiential observations which can enrich the conceptual system in the continuing search for systematic relationships among a range of phenomena. Concomitantly, it must be kept in mind that "the accuracy of an observation does not, in itself, make it valuable to science."[1]

A conceptual system is characterized by an interrelated set of postulates having relevance for some central phenomenon. Out of the conceptual system, theories emerge directed toward achieving further understanding of the real world. Theories are abstractions. They underlie the development of testable hypotheses and, in the testing, may be supported or refuted.

Every scientific statement does not have to be tested before it is accepted, but it must be capable of being tested.[2] History provides many examples of notions found highly useful long before being subjected to experiential verification. This is not to propose that testing may not be necessary, but rather to point out that theories may be quite significant even before they have been tested. The generation of theory is the outgrowth of abstract thought and abstraction is clearly different from concrete behavior. The formulation of theories is concerned with relationships. The capacity to envision new ways of perceiving phenomena and to propose meaningful explanations for these perceptions is a characteristic of theoretical formulation. "Observation and experiment do not provide the conceptions without which inquiry is aimless and blind."[3]

The emergence of a science of nursing demands a clear, unequivocal conceptual frame of reference. This is not to propose that nursing's conceptual system is either static or inflexible. Quite the contrary. In its evolution it is properly subject to reformulation and change as empirical knowledge grows, as conceptual data achieve greater clarity, and as the interconnectedness between ideas takes on new dimensions. Nursing's abstract system is a matrix of concepts relevant to the life process in man. Postulates integral to the system are asserted and testable hypotheses derive from the system.

Nursing is an empirical science. As with other empirical sciences, its purpose is to describe and explain the phenomenon central to its concern and to predict about it. The life process in man is a phenomenon of wholeness, of continuity, of dynamic and creative change. The multiplicity of events, both actual and potential, that may attend its becoming provide the experiential data of nursing research. The identification of relationships between events provides for an ordering of knowledges and for the development of nursing's hypothetical generalizations and unifying principles.

If the process of life is to be studied and understood, normal and pathological processes must be treated on a basis of complete equality. Health and illness, ease and dis-ease are dichotomous notions, arbitrarily defined, culturally infused, and value laden. The life process possesses its own unity. It is inseparable from the environment. The characteristics of the life process are those of the whole. As the life process in man is understood, its multiple manifestations lend themselves to explanation and to prediction.

A concept of the life process in man that views the notions of normal and pathological as invalid bases for studying man may not be readily perceived by those who have been imbued with the idea that health and sickness are discrete entities, each subject to its own independent study. But health and sickness, however defined, are expressions of the process of life. Whatever meaning they may have is derived out of an understanding of the life process in its totality. Life's deviant course demands that it be viewed in all of its dimensions if valid explanations of its varied manifestations are to emerge. Predictions, the keys to knowledgeable intervention, will be no better than the extent to which they arise out of an increasing understanding of life's innumerable potentialities.

The all-too-common perception of man as predominantly subjected to multiple negative environmental influences with pathological outcomes denies man's unity with nature and his evolutionary becoming. A man-environment dichotomy is presumed, rather than recognition of the complementary nature of the man-environment relationship. The well documented negentropic qualities of life require a positive approach for their understanding.

The development of a science brings with it the need for a language of specificity.[4] The language of everyday life is filled with ambiguities. The word "field" may be used to refer to a cotton field, a baseball field, a magnetic field, an airport, or a sphere of influence. For one person the word "nuts" may conjure up visions of an edible delight while for another there may arise an image of small metal blocks with threaded holes in them. To someone else "nuts" may represent an exclamation of disgust or scorn. Semantic confusion is not an uncommon problem among people. Generally one determines the meaning of a word within the context of its usage and does not pursue exactness of meaning with the user. While this kind of generality seems to serve reasonably well for much of day-to-day living, it is highly inadequate for scientific use.

The development of a scientific language evolves out of the general language. Terms in everyday usage are given precise and unambiguous meanings. They are then so understood by all members of a given scientific discipline. Development of such a language is directed toward achieving simplicity and clarity. Depiction of reality attains greater accuracy. Symbolic representation of relationships becomes possible. On occasion it may be necessary to invent a new word in order to secure adequate precision and clarity. That a new word may have to be coined is not a "carte blanche" for a rash of new terminology. Nor is a scientific language properly developed for the purpose of covering up a pseudoscientism (not an unheard-of feat). Jargon, one of Langer's[5] "Idols of the Laboratory," is more of a pretense toward technical sophistication than it is an expression of ideas.

Description, stated in general language terms, attends the early stages of development of a science. With growth of a particular science, there arises the need for more precise terminology in which to state generalizations and to communicate the abstract formulations of the science. The furtherance of scientific inquiry in nursing requires a technical language of specificity. Translation of nursing's body of scientific knowledge into meaningful service to man demands that explanatory and predictive principles possess clarity and exactness.

Nursing aims to assist people in achieving their maximum health potential. Maintenance and promotion of health, prevention of disease, nursing diagnosis, intervention, and rehabilitation encompass the scope of nursing's goals. Nursing is concerned with people—all people—well and sick, rich and poor, young and old. The arenas of nursing's services extend into all areas where there are people: at home, at school, at work, at play; in hospital, nursing home, and clinic; on this planet and now moving into outer space.

The science of nursing aims to provide a body of abstract knowledge growing out of scientific research and logical analysis and capable of being translated into nursing practice. Nursing's body of scientific knowledge is a new product specific to nursing.

Concomitantly, the science of nursing does not arise out of a vacuum nor are the knowledges encompassed by nursing science necessarily of meaning only to nurses.

Nursing is a humanistic science. As such, the methods of classical science have a number of limitations for applicability to nursing research. Reductionism, representative of an atomistic world view in which complex things are built up of simple elements, is contrary to a perception of wholeness. The subjective world of human feelings must be incorporated into so-called "objective science" to provide a more comprehensive epistemology relevant to the study of man. Dubos has written: "Science does not progress only by inductive, analytical knowledge. The imaginative speculations of the mind come first, the verification and the analytic breakdown come only later. And imagination depends upon a state of emotional and intellectual freedom which makes the mind receptive to the impressions that it receives from the world in its confusing, overpowering, but enriching totality."[6]

Maslow[7] decries what he calls desacralization of science and points out "that 'cool' perceiving and neutral thinking" are not the only ways for discovering truth. Such experiences as pain, joy, redness, etc., create major difficulties for investigators seeking "rigorous definition" as a method of concept formation. Peering through a microscope is deemed an acceptable means for securing objective knowledge, but one must question the validity of human beings as proper subjects for microscopic detachment. The real world encompasses observer and observed, with both contributing their measure to any ascribed situation. New methodologies must be devised to supplement, enhance, and transcend traditional approaches to the search for understanding.

A body of scientific knowledge is clearly different from the uses to which that knowledge may be put. The science of nursing is prerequisite to the process of nursing. The science of nursing must be incorporated into nursing's instructional programs. Concomitantly, students must have opportunity to test the validity and reliability of theory in the real situation—the laboratory of human life. Broad principles are put together in novel ways to help explain a wide range of events and multiplicity of individual differences. Action, based on predictions arising out of intellectual skill in the merging of scientific principles, becomes underwritten by intellectual judgments. The distinctive nature of professional practice in nursing is spelled out in nursing's unifying principles and hypothetical generalizations.

The education of professional practitioners in nursing requires the transmission of a body of scientific knowledge specific to nursing. This body of knowledge determines the safety and scope of nursing practice. The imaginative and creative use of knowledge for the betterment of man finds expression in the art of nursing. Education opens the doorway to developing the art of practice. The purpose of professional education is to provide the knowledge and tools whereby an individual may become an artist in his field. It is not to prepare the skilled practitioner. And as Robert Hutchins has noted, ". . . the most practical education is the most theoretical one."[8]

Nursing's abstract system is the outgrowth of concern for human health and welfare. The science of nursing aims to provide a growing body of theoretical knowledge whereby nursing practice can achieve new levels of meaningful service to man. A conceptual model of man is at the base of nursing's abstract system and provides a frame of reference from which guiding principles may be derived.

FOOTNOTES

1. Polanyi, Michael, *Personal Knowledge,* Chicago: The University of Chicago Press, 1958, p. 136.

2. Popper, Karl R., *The Logic of Scientific Discovery,* New York: Harper Torchbooks, 1965, p. 48.

3. Nagel, Ernest, "The Philosopher Looks at Science," *Medicine and the Other Disciplines.* New York: International Universities Press, Inc., 1960, p. 24.

4. Hempel, Carl G., *Fundamentals of Concept Formation in Empirical Science,* Chicago: University of Chicago Press, 1952, p. 1.

5. Langer, Susan, *Mind: An Essay on Human Feeling, Volume I,* Baltimore: The Johns Hopkins Press, 1967, p. 36.

6. Dubos, René, *The Dreams of Reason,* New York: Columbia University Press, 1961, p. 122.

7. Maslow, Abraham H., *The Psychology of Science,* New York: Harper and Row, 1966, p. 121.

8. Hutchins, Robert M., *The Learning Society,* New York: Frederick A. Praeger, Publishers, 1968, p. 8.

CHAPTER 12

NURSING'S CONCEPTUAL MODEL

> ". . . . the molding of a system of concepts means
> nothing less than the creation of a new language, a
> new mode of thinking."
>
> —F. Waismann

A system has been defined as "an assemblage of facts or ideas that is adjusted and regulated to form a connected whole."[1] The interrelatedness of ideas that gives wholeness and unity to nursing's conceptual system is built around the life process in man. As ideas become organized into a meaningful frame of reference, there emerges a conceptual model of the life process in man, which can then provide a base for theoretical operations pertinent to continuing study and elaboration of the conceptual system.

A conceptual model is an abstraction. Such a model is not real but is instead a *representation* of the universe or some portion thereof. A model of the life process in man is an imaginary construct which provides a way of perceiving the life process and serves as an aid to thinking. Revision and change occur as emerging empirical evidence points up inconsistencies and inadequacies in the proposed model. The theoretical nature of the model does not free it of the need to take into account the real world. Concomitantly, it is in the abstractness of the model that facts and observations are transcended and meaning emerges.

For purposes of this chapter, the terms "man," "life process," and "life process in man" are used interchangeably. "Model" is used to mean a "conceptual model of the life process in man." The model to be proposed represents a matrix of ideas which in its wholeness symbolizes man. Moreover, man is an integral part of the universe. Man and environment are complementary systems, *not* dichotomous ones. In consequence a model of man must affirm the unity of nature.

Nursing's conceptual model rests upon a set of basic assumptions which have been discussed in Unit II. These assumptions constitute statements of fact postulated to be true and describe the life process in man as characterized by wholeness, openness, unidirectionality, pattern and organization, sentience and thought. These are characteristics that underlie and must be taken into account in the development of the model.

An energy field identifies the conceptual boundaries of man. This field is electrical in nature, is in a continual state of flux, and varies continuously in its intensity, density, and extent. It may be likened to fields of the physical world in its capacity to demonstrate the presence of electrical charges and their correlates. Theoretically, electrical fields extend to infinity. Concomitantly, for practical purposes they may be deemed bounded according to selected criteria. The human field is postulated to have its boundary contiguous with the boundary of the environment. The environment is, itself, an energy field electrical in nature. The interaction between the human field and the environmental field takes place across the conceptual boundaries of these two fields which together are coextensive with the universe.

The human field extends beyond the discernible mass which we perceive as man. The concentration of energy, having a nature and density which is visible to the human eye, encompasses only a portion of an individual's identity. Multiple irregularities characterize the boundaries of man's energy field. At times the field may extend farther into the environment and at other times retreat in the direction of man's visible core. The nature and intensity of the man-environment interchange across these fluctuating boundaries varies both between individuals and for given individuals at different points in time.

Numerous colloquialisms suggest corollaries between such postulated energy fields and the observed world. For example, persons may be referred to as magnetic, forceful, moody, withdrawn—observations consistent with a concept of fluctuating field intensities and dimensions. The great actor, with capacity to enthrall an audience, penetrates the environmental boundary and his energy field, like a giant pseudopodium, reaches out to engulf a portion of the outer world, receding only when the drama ends.

The human field possesses its own identifiable wholeness. Despite its dynamic nature and its continuous interaction with the environment, it maintains identity in its ever-changing but omnipresent patterning. Pattern and organization of the field express themselves in a wide range of ways, all of which have relevance for the integrity of the field. Pattern evolves with kaleidoscopic uncertainty coordinate with the nature of the man-environment energy exchange taking place through space-time. Growing complexity of organization is an outgrowth of the multiple interactions occurring along the continuum of life. When pattern and organization no longer exist, the integrity of the human field is destroyed and death ensues.

Death is postulated to represent a transformation of energy. In whatever way one may perceive events subsequent to death, relevant testable hypotheses are yet to be proposed. At the same time, the passing of a human life has its own objective reality. At death the human field ceases to exist, and identity as a living human being is gone. The process of dying may be of long or short duration. It is a period of transition in which the integrity of the human field, as such, diminishes and dies.

Envision the human field embedded in the curvature of space-time. The life process is the expression of the rhythmical evolution of the field along a spiralling longitudinal axis, bound in the four-dimensional space-time matrix and ever shaping and being shaped by the environment. The human field occupies space, extending in all directions. The field projects into the future as well as into the past. The creativity of life emerges out of the man-environment interaction along life's continuum. The human field is continually adding new dimensions of growing complexity, evidenced in life's negentropic qualities.

The communication of concepts is sometimes helped by the use of concrete illustrations. The reader is no doubt familiar with the child's toy known as "Slinky." (There is also a "Junior Slinky" —smaller but perhaps more effective as an aid to understanding the proposed model). The life process lacks the evenness and regularity of this interesting toy, but with a little effort the "Junior Slinky" can be twisted, its spirals stretched or shortened, its intervals between spirals narrowed or widened. Larger spirals of "Slinky," itself, may be superimposed upon the spirals of the toy. Visualize "Slinky" as embedded in space and its sequence of spirals as coordinate with the passing of time.

Imagine the life process moving along the "Slinky" spirals with the human field occupying space along the spiral and extending out in all directions from any given location along a spiral.

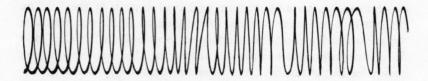

Each turn of the spiral exemplifies the rhythmical nature of life, while distortions of the spiral portray deviations from nature's regularities. Variations in the speed of change through time may be perceived by narrowing or widening the distance between spirals. (For example, compare 20 turns of the wire per inch to 5 turns per inch.) Energy exchange between the human field and environment is a constant concomitant of the evolving life process. Sentience and thought arise out of this interaction and give further evidence of the wondrousness of life. This is not to be interpreted as a mechanistic design. Rather, it is proposed as an aid to perceiving life's realities and potentialities.

The limitations of a concrete example to illustrate an abstraction are multiple. "Slinky" is proposed as a stimulus to ways of perceiving man. It is not a representation of man. The basic assumptions presented in Unit II underlie any extrapolation of ideas emerging out of examination of "Slinky." Nursing's conceptual model derives from a synthesis of ideas which then form a unified and meaningful system.

Man is a unified whole having his own distinctive characteristics which cannot be perceived by looking at or describing the parts. Nor does a summation of parts add up to man. The fundamental unit of the living system is an energy field. It is this field which gives unity to the concept of wholeness. The human field interacts as a whole with the whole of the environment. Changes taking place in the human field and in the environment are holistic in nature. Pattern and organization give identity to the field and are themselves field phenomena. Alterations in pattern and organization are continuous and reflect the unitary nature of the life process. Man evolves as a totality.

The most difficult construct to comprehend in nursing's conceptual model appears to be that concerning the wholeness of man. When man is perceived, the parts, whether cells, organs, or systems; biological, physical, or psychological; disappear from view. The whole and the parts cannot be perceived simultaneously.* The identity of man exists only in his wholeness. This wholeness is central and indispensable to nursing's conceptual model.

The life process is an evolutionary emergent. The capacity of life forms to transcend themselves is an expression of the advancing differentiation and complexity which characterizes both man and environment in their concomitant and interrelated evolution through space-time. The life process evolves along the curvature of space-time. Events along the continuum are unique. Events do not come again or repeat themselves. Similarity between events cannot be construed as repetition of events. Human behavior does not revert back to earlier stages—the path of life is undirectional.

Sentience and thought arise out of life's complexifying, probabilistic goal-directedness. Consciousness is a facet of man's becoming and in its emergence reflects man's expanding awareness of the world about him. In the process of evolution, man's search for meaning takes on new dimensions and his capacity for understanding grows. Ontogenesis and phylogenesis evidence a lengthening of conscious awareness (the waking state) through time. Coming into awareness is postulated to represent new levels of complexity with correlates in the ongoing development of cognition and feelings. The capacity to experience one's self and the world and to make sense out of one's experiences is an emergent along life's longitudinal axis.

Human behavior is synergistic.† Behavioral manifestations of the life process are symphonic expressions of unity and cannot be dichotomized as objective or subjective, as internal or external, as mental or physical. They are unique to the whole and their identification in the real world provides evidence of consistency in the interrelatedness of ideas which form the structure of nursing's conceptual model.

The model of the life process in man basic to nursing's abstract system may be postulated to be represented by an energy field embedded in the four-dimensional space-time matrix and becoming increasingly complex as it evolves rhythmically along life's longitudinal axis. Pattern and organization are maintained amidst

---

* The reader may wish to refer back to Chapter 6.

† Synergy is defined as the unique behavior of whole systems, unpredicted by any behaviors of their component functions taken separately.

the constant change attending the continuous interaction between man and environment. Nursing's principles of homeodynamics, discussed in the next chapter, derive from this model.

FOOTNOTES

1. Stulman, Julius, *Fields Within Fields Within Fields*, New York: The World Institute, Vol. 1, No. 1, Spring 1968, p. 7.

CHAPTER 13

HOMEODYNAMICS: PRINCIPLES OF NURSING SCIENCE

"... the existence of harmonies which foreshadow an indeterminate range of future discoveries."

—Michael Polanyi

Descriptive, explanatory, and predictive principles give substance to nursing's conceptual system and make possible knowledgeable nursing practice. Principles derive from the imaginative synthesis of available data. General patterns and regularities characterizing the phenomenon under study are identified and provide a means for systematically anticipating future events.

Principles are stated as hypothetical generalizations and theories. They are provisional. The degree to which a principle approximates reality increases as confirmation grows and greater precision is attained. Supplementation and modification of a principle may become necessary in order to encompass exceptions and to more faithfully represent the real world. To the extent that a principle possesses universality, its potential for usefulness increases.

Formulation of a principle opens the way to a range of investigations of conditions under which a particular principle holds. As evidence of the validity and reliability of a principle accumulates, its value as an empirical tool is enhanced. Commonalities between events come into view. The significance of a principle may take on new dimensions of meaning beyond those envisioned by the formulator of the principle. Principles are symbolic. They are representations of the real world and must be tested against actuality to verify their correctness.

The formulation of scientific principles basic to nursing derives from the conceptual model discussed in Chapter 12. Facts and ideas are synthesized to present a coherent pattern consistent with the known world. Unifying principles are proposed and are stated as hypothetical generalizations about the life process in man.

The life process is homeodynamic. An energy field, the fundamental unit of the living system, portrays the dynamic nature of life and is basic to the derivation of nursing science principles. The principles of homeodynamics enunciated and discussed in this chapter are four in number, namely: principle of *reciprocy*, principle of *synchrony*, principle of *helicy*, and principle of *resonancy*. These principles postulate the way the life process is and predict the nature of its evolving. These are broad generalizations which are deemed to conform to experiential data and to lay a foundation for developing testable hypotheses potentially fruitful in furthering nursing's understanding of the life process in man.

The theoretical basis of nursing is expressed in its guiding principles. Thus, the establishment of connections between events is made possible and technological application is permitted. Future occurrences are subject to prediction, and intervention directed toward achieving specified changes becomes practicable.

Fundamental principles are properly characterized by generality and precision. Description, couched in everyday language, may serve in the early stages of development of a science. However, explanatory and predictive effectiveness requires the evolving of a language of specificity with potential for symbolic and mathematical representations. Definitions take on increasing clarity and exactness.

A principle is a theoretical formulation. Facts, like pieces of a jigsaw puzzle, fall into place and achieve meaning within the framework of theory. Nursing's principles of homeodynamics provide a way for describing, explaining, and predicting a wide range of events having direct relevance for the professional practice of nursing. Let us proceed to a discussion of these principles.

PRINCIPLE OF RECIPROCY

The principle of reciprocy is predicated upon the basic assumptions of wholeness and openness and the dynamic nature of the universe. The life process in man is deemed to be characterized by an energy field which then may be specifically identified as the human field. The environment is defined as all that which is external to a given human field and is thus stated to be the environmental field. The human field and the environmental field are continuously interacting with one another.

The relationship between the human field and the environmental field is one of constant mutual interaction and mutual change. The mutuality of the man-environment interaction process specifies that man and environment are to be perceived simultaneously. These are reciprocal systems in which molding and being molded are taking place in both systems at the same time. The concept embodied in this principle is contrary to an older view of man adapting to multiple environmental forces. Rather, it is the man-environment interaction process that portends the future, not the flexibility of man in adjusting to environmental changes. The human field and the environmental field are continuously repatterned. With each repatterning, subsequent interaction is revised and new patterning in both man and environment emerges.

This principle provides a basis for explaining the creativity of life. It furnishes a conceptual approach to understanding why all persons exposed to a given disease do not become ill. Unanticipated outcomes associated with extensive use of D.D.T., the unpredicted reversal in purportedly diminishing tuberculosis and venereal disease rates, and emergence of the "battered child syndrome" become less surprising when viewed from the perspective of reciprocy.

The principle of reciprocy postulates the inseparability of man and environment and predicts that sequential changes in the life process are continuous, probabilistic revisions occurring out of the interactions between man and environment.

This principle may be stated in symbolic form thus:

$$R = f \ (M_1 \rightleftarrows E_1)$$

in which R stands for Reciprocy

M stands for the human field

E stands for the environmental field

and can be read as: "Reciprocy is a function of the mutual interaction between the human field and the environmental field."

PRINCIPLE OF SYNCHRONY

The principle of synchrony may be stated as follows: Change in the human field depends only upon the state of the human field and the simultaneous state of the environmental field at any given point in space-time.

The life process evolves unidirectionally along the space-time continuum and is bound in the four-dimensional space-time matrix. Space-time binding enunciates the contemporaneous nature of changes taking place between man and environment. The life process is a becoming. Developmental events along life's axis express the growing complexity of pattern and organization evolving out of multiple previous man-environment interactions. Each repatterning is a revision of the immediately preceding pattern. At each point in space-time, man is what he has been becoming but he is not what he has been. Moreover, he cannot go back to what he has been. Life proceeds unidirectionally and is inextricably bound within the space-time dimension.

Numerous and varied events attend the process of human development and are incorporated into ongoing developmental patterning and repatterning. Earlier developmental patterns are replaced by later ones. The particular pattern that identifies the human field at any given point in space-time is unique. The same is true for the environmental field. It is out of the simultaneous interaction between these two patterns that change occurs.

This principle neither denies nor ignores the reality of past events. The life process is a constantly evolving series of changes in which the past has been incorporated and out of which new patterns have emerged. This principle does place the past in a context of nonrepeatability and postulates that the determinants of change are only what man is at any given moment coupled with the state of the environment at the same moment.

This principle is in contradiction to an all-too-common practice of interpreting various behavioral manifestations in adults as equivalent to developmental behaviors occurring in an earlier developmental stage. Under this latter view, adults may be subjected to handling deemed appropriate to an earlier period, to the detriment of the individual.

Pattern and organization are basic to this principle. It is pattern which is revised in the man-environment interaction. Pattern and organization take on greater complexity as life evolves. Change reflects this dynamic repatterning and growing complexity.

This principle predicts that change in human behavior will be determined by the simultaneous interaction of the actual state of the human field and the actual state of the environmental field at any given point in space-time. Probable outcomes of this interaction encompass a range of possibilities some of which may be deemed more likely than others. Predictions of probable outcomes take on greater accuracy as means for determining and specifying states of the human and environmental fields achieve greater precision and as relationships between these states and subsequent events are established.

This principle may be stated in symbolic form thus:

$$S = f \ S\text{-}T_1 \ (M_1 \rightleftarrows E_1)$$

in which S stands for Synchrony

S-T stands for space-time

and can be read as: "Synchrony is a function of the state of the human field at a specified point in space-time interacting with the environmental field at the same specified point in space-time."

PRINCIPLE OF HELICY

The principle of helicy subsumes within it the principles of reciprocy and synchrony, and postulates further explanatory and predictive dimensions of nursing's theoretical system. The principle of helicy connotes that the life process evolves unidirectionally in sequential stages along a curve which has the same general shape all along but which does not lie in a plane. Encompassed within this principle are the concepts of rhythmicality, negentropic evolutionary emergence, and the unitary nature of the man-environment relationship.

The life process is characterized by probabilistic goal-directedness. Though the specific goal may not be known, increasing complexity of pattern and organization is a constant attendant of the developmental process. Man-environment interactions are directed toward achieving new dimensions of complexity. They are *not* directed toward achieving homeostasis or equilibrium (stable or un-

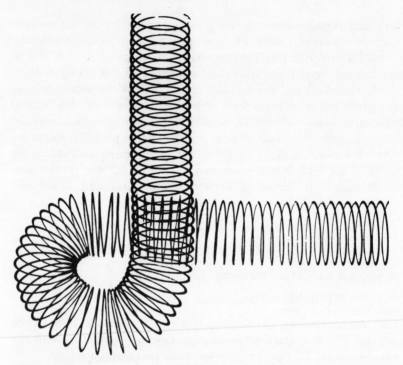

stable). The life process is continuously innovative and requires, for its understanding, a concept of man evolving.

Rhythmicalities portend probabilistic predictions. Life evolves along a spiralling longitudinal axis bound in the curvature of space-time. With each turn of the spiral along the axis, similarities appear. Spirals along the axis are further embedded within the spiralling of the axis itself (Figure 2). Rhythmic phenomena are expressions of the reciprocal relationship between man and environment. The rhythms of life are inextricably woven into the rhythms of the universe. Man and environment constitute a unitary whole.

The principle of helicy postulates an ordering of man's evolutionary emergence. The rise of cognition and feelings is encompassed. Predictive potential exists for a wide range of events in the real world. Cyclical similarities can be identified and probabilities determined. Earthbound man's advent into outer space and the bringing of extrasensory perception and other paranormal phenomena within the purview of recognized scientific endeavor are logical expressions of this principle.

This principle may be stated in symbolic form thus:

$$H = f \ S\text{-}T_1 \ (M_1 \rightleftarrows E_1) \, \underset{\sim}{i} \, f \ S\text{-}T_2 \ (M_2 \rightleftarrows E_2) \, \underset{\sim}{i} \text{-} f \ S\text{-}T_n \ (M_n \rightleftarrows E_n)$$

in which H stands for Helicy

    ⌇ stands for the spiral of life

    i stands for innovation

and can be read as: "Helicy is a function of continuous innovative change growing out of the mutual interaction of man and environment along a spiralling longitudinal axis bound in space-time."

PRINCIPLE OF RESONANCY

The principle of resonancy postulates that change in pattern and organization of the human field and the environmental field is propagated by waves. The life process in man is a symphony of rhythmical vibrations oscillating at various frequencies. Between man and environment there is a rhythmic flow of energy waves. An ordered arrangement of rhythms characterizes both the human field and the environmental field and undergoes continuous dynamic metamorphosis in the man-environment interaction process.

Man experiences his environment as a resonating wave of complex symmetry uniting him with the rest of the world. The life process may be likened to cadences—sometimes harmonic, sometimes cacophonous, sometimes dissonant; rising and falling; now fast, now slow—ever changing in a universal orchestration of dynamic wave patterns.

A multiplicity of waves characterizes the universe. Light waves, sound waves, thermal waves, atomic waves, gravity waves flow in rhythmic patterns—largely unseen, unheard, and unopen to man's capacity to see, hear, or perceive. The colorful auras of radiation waves surrounding radiating bodies are generally beyond the visible range of the human eye. These, and other waves, are integral facets of nature's rhythms.

The pattern of the human field is a wave phenomenon encompassing man in his entirety. The whole of man senses, feels, perceives, and reasons. Literary works speak of man swept by waves of grief or joy, loneliness, tenderness, and pain. The sick may "ache all over."

The resonance of change is a continuously propagating series of waves between man and environment, characterized by invariance under transformation. The predictive potentials of this principle arise out of a perception of the life process as an unending flow of wave patterns. The developmental process in growth of the individual is a good example of this principle.

PRINCIPLES OF HOMEODYNAMICS

The principles of homeodynamics postulate a way of perceiving unitary man. Changes in the life process in man are predicted to be inseparable from environmental changes and to reflect the mutual and simultaneous interaction between the two at any given point in space-time. Changes are irreversible, nonrepeatable. They are rhythmical in nature and evidence growing complexity of pattern and organization. Change proceeds by the continuous repatterning of both man and environment by resonating waves.

Evidence of conditions under which these principles hold arises out of examination of the real world. Investigations of a range of phenomena are necessary to provide the substantive data which can further the translation of these principles into practical application. Scientific research in nursing is beginning to underwrite the moving boundaries of nursing advances. Maintenance and promotion of health, disease prevention, diagnosis, intervention, and rehabilitation—nursing's goals—take on added dimensions as theoretical knowledge provides new direction to practice.

CHAPTER 14

VERIFICATION OF CONCEPTS

". . . . if the inquiry is well conceived it will not merely
come up with a new answer; it will come up with
something far more valuable, which is a new question,
one which had not been thought of before."

—J. Robert Oppenheimer

In what ways do the principles discussed in Chapter 13 find
verification in the real world? What evidence exists to support
these principles? What foundation has been laid to further the
elaboration of nursing's scientific base?

The science of nursing encompasses nursing's conceptual system. Basic research in nursing is directed toward advancing knowledge which can further understanding of man and his world.
There must be an advance before there can be application. Conceptual thought and theoretical inquiries are fundamental requi-
sites to the elaboration of nursing's body of abstract knowledge.
Basic research must underwrite applied research. Only then can
there be fruitful interaction between ideas and their translation
into human service.

Nursing's conceptual system provides a frame of reference in
which to lodge observations. The process of identifying meaningful
relationships between knowledges becomes possible. Cluster studies,
in which several investigators pursue different facets of a larger
question, provide a means whereby smaller truths may be integrated
to form a more fundamental truth.

Theoretical research in nursing is of relatively recent vintage.
Nonetheless, evidence is already beginning to acccumulate in support of the principles postulated in the previous chapter. Investigations into a range of human phenomena give substance to nursing's abstract system. Unexpected relationships, tangential to a
specific problem under investigation, may come into view. New

questions arise. Understanding grows. The basis for knowledgeable nursing practice is expanded.

An energy field was stated earlier to constitute the fundamental unit of a living system. This field is deemed a bounded whole possessing pattern and organization and undergoing continuous change in the interaction process between man and environment. The electrical nature of this field is well documented. Concomitantly, instrumentation capable of mapping the electrical boundaries of the human field and of providing indices of human field functioning have not been developed. Proposals that electrical correlates of cellular and subsystem performance might be extrapolated to the whole have not been substantiated.

Whether or not currently available instruments can be used to identify differentiating electrical indices of total human functioning is a question having high relevance for nursing. A series of studies based on the assumptions of wholeness and openness were designed to investigate the relationship between electrical potential differences, as measured by the Keithley Microvoltmeter, Model 153, and selected phenomena of the life process in man.

Two of the above-mentioned studies sought base line data that might be predictive of rhythmic changes occurring through time in normal populations. One[1] of these investigations measured electrical potential differences over a three-month period among normal adult females to determine whether or not ovulation would be reflected in the electrical potential difference readings. The other[2] (not yet completed) is concerned with investigating bioelectric potentials in nonpregnant and pregnant rabbits. In the latter instance, for practical reasons, New Zealand hares rather than human beings are being used as the study population. An investigation of electrical potential differences was carried out to test possible differences in readings between a normal adult male population and an adult male population of hemiplegics.[3] An additional study was done using suicidal patients as the comparative group.[4]

In none of these investigations have the electrical potential difference readings correlated with the variables under study. It would appear that the synergistic nature of the life process does not reveal itself in electrical potential differences as measured in these studies. One might raise a question concerning the studies of hemiplegics and suicidal patients as to whether there might have been differences had these two groups been under investigation at the onset or most acute period of their conditions. Other approaches or different instrumentation might perhaps yield useful data. Although the findings in the studies noted above do not support using voltmeter measurements to predict life process phenomena, various irregularities in the findings do support further investigation.

The complementary nature of the man-environment relationship and the growing complexity of life through time are evidenced in Mathwig's[5] investigation. Dr. Mathwig used Sprague-Dawley albino rats representing an age span of 56 to 500 days (puberty through the aging adult in rats) to determine temporal relationships between selected living system variables and selected environmental variables. Her findings provide empirical evidence in support of the principles of homeodynamics.

Today's enthusiasm for jogging grew out of reported relationships between physical exercise and selected facets of physiological functioning. However, the possibility that motion might have a significant bearing on the nature and speed of the developmental process is an idea of a very different order. Nursing's conceptual model postulates a complexifying life process characterized by a continuously changing energy field. What might be the effect of increasing the motion of this already dynamic field? Might ordering and reordering of the human field proceed with greater speed and coherence in the presence of environmentally induced motion?

The findings of three studies support a significant relationship between imposed motion and infant growth and development. Neal,[6] using a population of premature infants, demonstrated that subjects on a standardized regimen of motion showed significantly higher achievement ($P<.001$) on the motor and maturation scales of the Rosenblith "Behavioral Test for Neonates" than did subjects not on the motion regimen. Neal further notes that "Rosenblith has shown that the motor response score of this test has a definite relationship to activity level and mental development on the eighth-month assessment using the Bayley Test." The rocking regimen used by Neal was carried out from the fifth day of life to the 251st day following conception for all infants in the experimental group.

Porter[7] tested the effects of planned passive exercise on development with a study population of normal, full-term, 4- to 16-week-old infants. Gesell Developmental Schedules were used to compare the experimental and control groups before and after carrying out the exercise regimen. Experimental infants were exercised for two 10-minute periods daily, six days a week, for a period of two months. Both experimental and control groups received equivalent handling and emotional support throughout the study. At completion of the study period, the experimental group significantly exceeded the control group on all six criterion measures used, specifically: weight, $P < .006$; height, $P < .001$; motor, $P < .004$; adaptive, $P < .002$; language, $P < .0002$; and personal-social, $P < .0001$.

Findings similar to those of Neal and Porter are reported in Earle's[8] study of normal full-term neonates. Though Earle's findings are less definitive than those of Neal and Porter, they are nonetheless consistent. Earle studied three groups of infants according to (a) supplementary mechanical kinesthetic stimulation, (b) supplementary maternal kinesthetic stimulation, and (c) kinesthetic stimulation afforded by routine nursery care. Infants in Group (a) were rocked in a cradle whereas infants in Group (b) were held while being rocked in a rocking chair. Neonates on the rocking regimens were rocked for 30 minutes three times a day from six hours after birth through the third day of life. The Rosenblith test was used to determine developmental levels for the three groups of infants. Those infants receiving supplementary maternal kinesthetic stimulation achieved a significantly higher $(P < .05)$ developmental level than did infants on routine nursery care. The developmental level for infants receiving supplementary mechanical kinesthetic stimulation approached significance in comparison with infants on routine nursery care. The very short time period (3 days) to which Earle's infants were subjected to their motion regimen in comparison with Neal's (1 to 2 months) and Porter's (2 months) suggests that Earle might well have found statistical significance for her mechanically stimulated infants had she continued her regimen for a longer period of time.

A direct relationship between environmentally imposed motion and infant growth and development has been empirically validated. Might one go beyond these data and postulate a relationship between increased motion and a speeding up of creative evolution? In 1885 Harper's magazine carried an item that read in part: "Was he born on wheels? Was he cradled in a pullman? He has always been in motion probably; he was started at 30 miles an hour, no doubt, this marvellous boy of our new era. He was not born in a house at rest, but the locomotive snatched him along with a shriek and a roar before his eyes were fairly open, and he was rocked in a 'section', and his first sensation of life was that of moving rapidly over vast arid spaces, through cattle ranges, and along canyons. The effect of quick and easy locomotion on character may have been noted before but it seems that here is the production of a new sort of man, the direct product of our railway era. . . . He belongs to the new expansive race that must live in motion."[9]

In the last half-century man's exposure to motion has far exceeded that offered by the early locomotives. Automobiles, fast trains, airplanes, jet propulsion, and now supersonic travel, not to mention outer-space vehicles, have created an era of escalating acceleration for the human race. What developmental changes might today's accelerated motion portend for man? The principle of helicy provides a base for deriving testable hypotheses relevant to this question.

The effects of motion in influencing patterning and organization of the life process need further exploration. What kinds of motion might be postulated to be most effective in helping man to achieve maximum health? What is the nature of the organizing process by which the human field is oriented toward fulfilling its developmental potential?

Other environmental influences concerned with the development of the life process have also undergone investigation. Downs[10] studied the relationship between maternal stress and fetal development. Infants born to mothers experiencing stress during pregnancy, as operationally defined in this study (i.e., major geographical moves, changes in family structure, family strife, death in family, illness in family, marital infidelity, desertion by father, loss of financial security, etc.), had a significantly higher $(P < .02)$ incidence of neonatal pathology than did infants born to mothers who had not experienced such stresses. The empirical evidence is consistent with the principles of reciprocy and synchrony.

Fagin's[11] study of rooming-in for mothers of hospitalized children 1½ through 3 years of age not only supported the importance of the mother's presence in the hospital but suggested an unexpected dividend. Children whose mothers remained with them were significantly different $(P < .001)$ from children whose mothers did not remain in the hospital in reactions to temporary, brief separation from the mother, emotional dependence, appetite, food finickiness, and urine training, both at one week and at one month following hospitalization. The surprise came when it appeared that the developmental level of the children who had been hospitalized with their mothers present might possibly exceed that of nonhospitalized children.

Established regularities between a range of rhythmic variables are known to undergo revision as jet travelers, transported in one continuous journey across several time zones, change to follow the clock time in effect at their destination. Generally not considered, however, have been the possible effects of daylight-saving time on established regularities.

Felton[12] postulated that an abrupt one-hour change in social routines would be reflected in blood pressure and temperature readings. She found that the change to daylight-saving time, with its concomitant change in the environmental schedule, acted to modify the blood pressure and temperature cycles as if the subjects had moved rapidly through one or more time zones. Moreover, her data revealed that the time required for blood pressure readings to adjust to the new environmental time was two days whereas temperature readings did not become synchronized with the new clock time for five days after the onset of daylight-saving time.

What are the implications of Felton's findings for human functioning in the period immediately following the abrupt one-hour time change which occurs twice a year with daylight-saving time and which affects a total population? A common denominator between daylight-saving time, jet excursions, supersonic travel, and orbiting space ships might be postulated to be a significant variable in determining man's evolutionary future. On a very practical level, to what extent may contemporary hospital routines compromise human functioning at a point when such compromise may have potentially serious consequences?

Efforts to determine predictive indices associated with a range of man-environment events have provided empirical evidence of relationships between many variables. In instances in which hypotheses have been rejected, evidence has accrued indicating the need for further studies either of the original hypotheses or of new questions arising out of the findings of a given study.

Runnerstrom,[13] investigating the efficacy of adequate food iron intake versus ingestion of iron supplements in maintaining acceptable hemoglobin levels during pregnancy, encountered an

unanticipated number of pregnant women who were pica practitioners. In consequence, although her findings generally supported
her hypotheses, the need for further work in this area with persons
having very low hemoglobin levels was evident.

A study of pica practitioners carried out by Dunston[14] revealed
a far larger incidence of pica practice than had previously been
reported in the literature. Dunston found a significantly higher
(P < .01) incidence of prematurity and perinatal mortality among
pica practitioners than among non-pica practitioners, irrespective
of hemoglobin level.

It is noteworthy that both Runnerstrom and Dunston uncov-
ered a higher incidence of pica practice in their study populations
than is ordinarily thought to exist. What further investigations
need to be carried out to better understand the relationships between maternal dietary practices (normal and abnormal) and fetal
development? To what extent is hemoglobin level an adequate
index of maternal health?

Social class membership has been implicated as an environmental index of human behavior under various conditions.[15, 16,.
17, 18] Studied in conjunction with other variables, social class might
be proposed to have potentials for identifying relationships different from those attributed to social class alone. When viewed
within the context of environmental wholeness, class structure
becomes subsumed within the patterned complexity of a larger
dimension. Investigations from such a perspective are needed.

Only a few studies were selected for inclusion in this chapter
They were chosen to illustrate a range of empirical evidence
growing out of nursing research. When examined within the
framework of nursing's conceptual system, these investigations
further the development of substantive knowledge to underwrite
nursing practice. As additional research findings are fitted into
place, potentials for identifying new relationships increase. A range
of unrelated data in nursing has been accumulating. Its incorporation into nursing's abstract system is imperative.

FOOTNOTES

1. Kuhtik, Nellie, "Ovulation in White Females and Bioelectric Potential
Differences," unpublished Doctoral Dissertation, New York University Division
of Nurse Education, 1968.
2. Hazzard, Mary, "Bioelectric Potentials in Non-Pregnant and Pregnant
Rabbits," Doctoral Dissertation in progress, New York University Division of
Nurse Education.

3. Ramey, Irene, "Hemiplegia, Muscle Function, and Bioelectric Potential Differences," unpublished Doctoral Dissertation, New York University Division of Nurse Education, 1967.

4. Monck, Maureen, "Bioelectrical Potential Differences and Suicidal Behavior," unpublished Doctoral Dissertation, New York University Division of Nurse Education, 1967.

5. Mathwig, Gean, "Living, Open Systems, Reciprocal Adaptation and the Life Process," unpublished Doctoral Dissertation, New York University Division of Nurse Education, 1968.

6. Neal, Mary, "Vestibular Stimulation and Developmental Behavior of the Small Premature Infant," *Nursing Research Report,* New York: American Nurses Foundation, March 1968. Doctoral Dissertation, New York University Division of Nurse Education, 1967.

7. Porter, Luz, "Physical-Physiological Activity and Infants' Growth and Development," unpublished Doctoral Dissertation, New York University Division of Nurse Education, 1967.

8. Earle, Anne, "The Effect of Supplementary Post-Natal Kinesthetic Stimulation on the Developmental Behavior of the Normal Female Newborn," unpublished Doctoral Dissertation, New York University Division of Nurse Education, 1969.

9. *Harper's Centennial Issue,* Vol. 201, No. 1205, October 1950, p. 125.

10. Downs, Florence, "Maternal Stress in Primigravidas as a Factor in the Production of Neonatal Pathology," unpublished Doctoral Dissertation, New York University Division of Nurse Education, 1964.

11. Fagin, Claire, *Rooming-In and Its Effect on the Behavior of Young Children,* Philadelphia: F. A. Davis Company, 1966.

12. Felton, Geraldene, "An Abrupt One Hour Shift in the Social Routine and the Extent and Duration of Blood Pressure and Temperature Changes in Young Women," unpublished Doctoral Dissertation, New York University Division of Nurse Education, 1968.

13. Runnerstrom, Lillian, "Food Iron Intake and Hemoglobin Levels," unpublished Doctoral Dissertation, New York University Division of Nurse Education, 1963.

14. Dunston, Beverly N., "Pica, Hemoglobin, and Prematurity and Perinatal Mortality," unpublished Doctoral Dissertation, New York University Division of Nurse Education, 1961.

15. Kessler, Eunice, "Distress Among Mothers of Hospitalized Two Through Four Year Old Children and Its Relationship to Social Class Membership," unpublished Doctoral Dissertation, New York University Division of Nurse Education, 1968.

16. Krieger, Dolores, "Attitudes Toward Physically Deviant Behavior and Social Class Membership of Significant Persons, and Social Responsibility in the Cerebral Palsied Adult," unpublished Doctoral Dissertation, New York University Division of Nurse Education, 1967.

17. Palmer, Irene, "Perceptions of Patients to Imminent General Surgery," unpublished Doctoral Dissertation, New York University Division of Nurse Education, 1963.

18. Putnam, Phyllis, "Social Class and Interpersonal Interaction in Young Children," unpublished Doctoral Dissertation, New York University Division of Nurse Education, 1963.

CHAPTER **15**

FORMULATING TESTABLE HYPOTHESES

"What is demanded for the hypothesis first of all is that it explain what is unknown, that it conform to the data in hand. But what this amounts to is the seeing of a pattern and this is, in essence, a synthesizing act of the imagination."
—Harold K. Schilling

Nursing's professionally educated members carry a signal responsibility for the elaboration and substantiation of nursing's scientific base. Of major importance is the development of scholarly, theoretical research that probes the unknown and opens new gateways to understanding human beings and the world in which they live. At the same time, it is equally essential that all of nursing's baccalaureate and higher degree graduates be motivated by a compelling urge to further their own knowledge and to exploit this knowledge for the enhancement of nursing practice.

Deep-seated curiosity coupled with human compassion underwrites the need to know that mankind may benefit. The "whys" of human behavior and human endeavor, immersed within a universe of mystery and magnificence, must be sought diligently and with imagination. Only as the "whys" become understood can there be "hows" knowledgeably designed to achieve nursing's goals.

Nursing's conceptual model connotes a way of perceiving man. From this vantage point are derived testable hypotheses having relevance for nursing. It is this model which establishes the frame of reference for envisioning relationships between events. The ordering of facts takes place within the context of nursing's conceptual system and achieves meaning within this context.

This chapter is not designed to discuss the nature of concept formation nor to provide the reader with an introduction to methods of research. Rather, its purpose is to identify some significant questions and to propose potentially productive areas for investigation. Glenn Seaborg, in a paper presented to the Secondary Education Board Conference in 1957, compared "scientific research to mountain climbing in an unexplored range. Considerable preparation, training, and strong motivation is required to get up to the upper altitudes even if no one particular stretch of the way is particularly difficult, but once there, it is relatively easy for one to see vistas or even to stumble across new riches."[1]

To reach the upper altitudes requires the knowledge and tools implicit in doctoral study of stature. It further requires the capacity for imaginative synthesis of ideas and facts for new understandings. Concomitantly, the creative, intelligent, independent, curious, skeptical, energetic, nonconformist, professionally educated student or practitioner, emotionally committed to her career and possessing superior conceptual ability, is likely to carry within her the germ of creative research. She must be encouraged and at times tolerated so that she may one day fulfill her potential for advancing nursing knowledge.

The cycle of progress is maintained by fruitful interaction between the discovery of new knowledge and the application of that knowledge. Applied research in nursing must accompany basic research in nursing. Furthermore, there are a multitude of studies that can contribute substantial empirical evidence useful to nursing that properly fall within the purview of nursing's baccalaureate and master's degree graduates. The elaboration of nursing's knowledge base and its incorporation into the instructional process and practice areas are of critical importance.

A fundamental question needing exploration concerns the topology of the human field. The living system is an energy field postulated to be characterized by a fluctuating boundary coordinate with the boundary of the environmental field. How can the boundary of a human field be identified?

Man's conceptual boundary encompasses the totality of the human field, only a portion of which is visible to the human eye. Concomitantly, the electrical nature of this field supports a proposal for the identification of electrical correlates capable of delineating the boundary of a human field. To determine the aforesaid correlates requires that there be an operational definition of the human field and that there be valid and reliable measuring instruments. Means for identifying electrical fields already exist. The adaptation of existing technology and the development of new instrumentation capable of making human field measurements would seem a reasonable possibility.

The energy field of an individual is hypothesized to vary in size, shape, intensity, and density as life progresses from birth through old age and death. Base line data identifying variations in field boundaries associated with development and aging would make possible investigations of a wide range of factors that might be related to field variability. Outcomes of such studies could provide evidence of relationships having valuable predictive potential for nursing diagnosis and intervention in health and illness.

Means of determining electrical correlates of human field intensity and density would provide a further source of descriptive data about the life process in man. Here again base line data are needed in order to determine correlates of human field variability according to the dimensions of field intensity and density. Determination of predictable interrelationships between human field size, shape, intensity, and density could lead to identification of indices having evaluative and interventional significance.

Other approaches to the study of human field boundaries must be explored. Where does the individual perceive his boundary to be? What are some implications of differences that may occur between an individual's perceived boundary and his visible mass which is identified as physical man? In what ways and under what conditions do perceptual boundaries vary in size and shape? What does a person mean when he says, "I feel expansive" or "I shrink when I see so-and-so"? Do such comments reflect changing energy field dimensions? The developing child is noted to go through an "I, me, mine" stage. Could this be an expression of growing coherence of the human field out of which conscious identity of self emerges? Do human field boundaries take on increased definitiveness in the process of growth?

Human beings are radiation bodies. The capacity of some persons to perceive radiation phenomena emanating from individuals has been reported extensively in the literature over many years. The subjective nature of such observations, difficulties encountered in efforts to validate the reality of these phenomena, and a general tendency to deny the existence of occurrences not within the visual capabilities of many people are problems. Descriptive data in this area could make a significant contribution to advancing knowledge about man's energy field.

Effects of imposed motion on developmental patterns in premature and full-term infants were reported in the preceding chapter. Do similar relationships exist throughout the life span? Is motion a significant factor in man's patterning and organization? Could there be a relationship between the nature and speed of motion and the coherence and integrity of the individual? Is motion an integrating force? How might motion be related to such factors as longevity and rhythmic phenomena? Answers to these and other questions could provide important guidelines for nursing practice.

The dynamic nature of man and environment specifies a world in motion. Life's negentropic qualities portend innovation and growing complexity. How may motion be related to increased ontogenetic and phylogenetic complexification.

Folklore, literature, and science attribute a range of human responses to a wide variety of sounds. Modern technology and urban living have added a new dimension to sonic phenomena. The environmental sound pattern has become more complex. What is the nature of the relationship between sound patterns and developmental processes? How are sound waves related to pattern formation and transformation of the human field?

Not all sonic phenomena are audible to the human ear, but they are all, nonetheless, active ingredients in the man-environment interaction process. Out of the merging of a multiplicity of sound waves, audible and inaudible, there arises a new product. It is this product that requires investigation. Are there identifiable correlates of sonic patterns that can be used to predict human behavior? Is there an association between the nature and speed of sound and the nature and speed of the aging process?

Man's capacity to communicate with man by other than the traditional five senses is a puzzle of long standing. That such events do take place has considerable word-of-mouth support. The means whereby such communication occurs and an understanding of the process involved are subjects of much conjecture. Are normally inaudible sound waves involved? Is this a radiation phenomenon having similarity to the visible radiation perceived by some people? Is such communication a further expression of man's emerging consciousness? What are the natures of the human field pattern and the simultaneous environmental field pattern that are coincident with thought transmission by extrasensory means? Are there identifiable field correlates of thought transmission?

Teen-age discotheques have been implicated in hearing problems among young people exposed to the high-volume noise levels common to such places. Loudness, whether on radio, record player, stereo set, or television, is commonly sought by the contemporary adolescent. Musical patterns popular today are quite different from those of even a generation back. Transistor radios and their ear button attachments are accepted accouterments of youth on streets and buses, at school and at home. What is signified by this extensive exposure to oft-heard selected sound patterns in adolescent development? What part does sound volume play in orientation of the human field? What is the relationship between environmental sound rhythms and the rhythms of the individual? What feelings are evoked that may have relevance for mankind's evolving?

Awareness of the passage of time is a long-standing concomitant of the human condition. In the real world of physical events, clock time is used to define time duration. However, time perception may vary noticeably from clock time, with a range of variables proposed as correlates of such variations. Age differences, thermal and biochemical factors, occupational involvement, and sleep-wake states are some of the areas that have been implicated in efforts to explain time perception variations. Is time perception a reflection of the real world or is it a deviation from the real world? Can it be that time perception is a relative reality?

Persons report perceptions of time flying, of time dragging, of time standing still, of timelessness. Inconsistencies between estimates of time duration and clock time are not uncommon. Is the speed with which time is perceived to be passing an index of the speed with which the aging process is occurring? What is the nature of the relationship between time perception and the integrity of the human field? Is perception of the passing of time a rhythmical phenomenon? Are there electrical correlates of time perception that can be identified? What kind of relationships exist between time perception and sensory phenomena? Do persons who evidence extrasensory perception perceive the passing of time differently from those who do not evidence such experiences?

The human field is embedded in a four-dimensional space-time matrix with the human field boundaries continuously changing in the process of life. The human field may then be postulated to occupy the dimension of space-time, thus incorporating facets of both man's past and future. The concept of present takes on an enlarged meaning. How are pattern and organization emerging out of the man-environment interaction process associated with the nature and extent of the human field and the capacity of an individual to remember the past and to envision the future? Are there unrecognized developmental dimensions and rhythmical phenomena hidden within the space-time continuum?

The capacity for memory and vision vary both within and between individuals along life's axis. Are retrocognition and precognition facets of this phenomenon? What environmental configurations may be associated with memory and vision? Are indices to be found in cosmic phenomena; in thermal, biochemical, or radiation factors; in the nature and speed of the man-environment interaction; in ontogenetic and phylogenetic rhythms; in interchange between living systems? Can human field boundaries be identified within the space-time dimension?

A view of time and space as separate dimensions, each worthy of investigation in its own right, has grown in recent years. Some questions relating to time have already been raised. What is the meaning of space? How does man perceive space? Effects of overcrowding among animal populations has received considerable attention. The significance of personal space and its relationship to various behavioral manifestations is under investigation. Population density has been associated with a range of social and anti-social activities. What are the environmental space needs of people? How may these vary between individuals? What indices may be used to predict space needs? How may environmental field and human field density and intensity be related to changing space needs? How is the nature of environmental space related to the developmental potential of the individual and of man? Is space perception a relative reality?

From Malthus to the present, man has evidenced growing concern with increasing numbers in the population. Today's "population explosion" has set in motion world-wide efforts to control fertility and to limit the number of births. That population growth seems to have rhythmical correlates is observable in life tables that extend over several generations. Ecological factors are admittedly recognized as playing a role in the nature and extent of fertility potential. Biochemical correlates of human fertility find expression in the widespread popularity of the "birth control pill." Detrimental outcomes are being postulated by investigators of the genetic effects of L.S.D. and similar drugs. More recently D.D.T. has been implicated as a possibly significant factor in fertility. The effects of thalidomide and German measles on embryonic development are immediate and well known.

Massive and rapid ecological shifts associated with a wide range of biochemical innovations need not be immediately observable to be nonetheless significant. Probabilistic evolution has a range of potential outcomes. The changes taking place in the human race will not be measured in mortality rates but rather in the capacity of life forms to transcend themselves. How may the "pill" and other drugs be affecting the long-range potentials of human development? Are there identifiable correlates already in evidence? Are there predictive indices having relevance for man's daily life? Does the mushrooming population growth portend the next development in man, providing an ample source from which progenitors of the future may emerge?

Investigations of a wide range of rhythmic phenomena have multiplied in recent years. Evidence of rhythmic relationships between environmental and biological factors is well documented. Phase relationships between biological system and subsytsem components are demonstrable. The significance of rhythmicalities as a basis for probabilistic predictions is high.

It has been postulated earlier that man-environment rhythmicalities portend evolutionary emergence—the increasing creative complexity of life. How might the sleep-wake cycle be viewed within this context. Ontogenetically, the individual begins life by sleeping the major portion of each 24-hour period. As the developmental process evolves, the sleep-wake ratio becomes reversed and the adult is awake the major portion of each 24-hour period. In the history of man, an analogous evolutionary process may be observed.

Can there be a relationship between man's rousing awareness and today's accelerating change? Do social vision and the search

for meaning have correlates in an enlarged capacity for viewing man's place in the natural world? Is there a relationship
between the dreams of sleep and "day-dreams"? Is there meaning
to be found in the dreaming (?) that occurs in that little-under-
stood state between sleeping and waking? Does the sleep-wake
rhythm reflect a facet of the space-time dimension? Are there patterns of variability in sleep-wake rhythms that correlate with health
and illness, with the process of aging, with developmental patterns?

Life's rhythms are integral to and inseparable from environmental rhythms. Deviations in the rhythmical relationship between
man and environment may be postulated to manifest themselves in
disruption and reorganization of the human field and the environmental field directed toward evolving a new rhythmical relationship between man and environment. What is the significance of the
disruption process? How does disruption affect the integrity of the
human field? What is the relationship between disrupted rhythms
and human illness? What factors may be associated with the nature
of an individual's response to rhythmic disruption?

Man is prone to claim control over various portions of his
environment when in reality he rearranges his environment in hopes
that the results will be in accord with some predetermined goal. Too
often man's rearranging is rooted in shortsightedness and narrow
vision. Immediate goals may seem to be achieved at the same time
that man unwittingly sets in motion unanticipated changes of far
greater significance. Substituting multiple causation for single
causation has contributed little to an enlarged perspective of the
nature of change or of man-environment interaction phenomena.
Rather, the holistic nature of man and his environment and the
reciprocal relationship between the two find expression in the
continuous repatterning of both, and portend the future.

How may environmental patterns be identified? How may
human field patterning be described? Are there observational indices of patterning that may have predictive potential? Does human
field patterning have postural correlates, or electrical correlates, or
sensory correlates? What is the nature of the repatterning process?
What is man's capacity for conscious participation in repatterning
the human field and the environment?

A large portion of daily life is currently hedged with "don'ts"
as investigators purport to find pathology burgeoning in association

with such things as cholesterol levels, cigarette smoking, sugar sub-
stitutes, radiation levels, sedentary habits, automobile exhaust
fumes, pesticides, drugs, water and air pollution, overeating, and a
vast number of other factors. Large sums of money are invested
annually to train personnel and to treat the "emotionally ill" while
at the same time automation, big business, complex governments,
and proponents of a mechanistic definition of life further deperson-
alize the individual. Economically, educationally, and socially deprived groups struggle for opportunity and recognition while vested
interests endeavor to maintain an obsolete hierarchal control. Upheaval takes place on college campuses while Vista and Peace Corps
volunteers seek to serve the less fortunate. Man walks upon the
moon.

How might the events mentioned in the previous paragraph be
interpreted according to nursing's principles of homeodynamics?
Might one propose that these events are part of the configuration
of escalating changes taking place today? May they not be expressions of evolutionary progression? Are the widespread, fear-inducing
(and often contradictory) "don'ts" valid bases for action or are they
artifacts parading as indices of the life process in man? Are there
identifiable patterns in apparent discrepancies and dichotomies that
can provide clues to a better understanding of the life process in
man? How are contemporary events expressive of the sequential
and creative nature of life?

In a world beset with wars and rumors of wars, where neighbor
attacks neighbor, and parental child abuse has become so marked
as to lead to legislative controls, when adolescent gangs roam the
streets with switchblades in hand, and hierarchal systems—whether
racial, governmental, economic, social, etc.—are in turmoil as demands for human rights take on increasingly militant expressions,
one may properly question ecological relationships which might
portend hostility, anger, fear, aggression, and repression, etc., as
probabilistic outcomes and those ecological factors which might
presage respect for human dignity, freedom, acceptance of individual and group differences, love, etc.

So-called pathological conditions, whatever their nature and
their overt manifestations, are probabilistic expressions of man-environment interaction and unidirectional transition. What are the
implications then for interpreting disease incidence, distribution,

susceptibility, prognosis, and seemingly causal factors coupled with anatomical, biological, sociocultural, psychological and physical, etc., deviations occurring within the context of holistic patterning?

The search for understanding of man and his world has barely begun. Multiple questions wait to be answered. New relationships must be envisioned and tested. As new knowledge comes into view, older ideas will be revised. Resynthesis of knowledges will reveal new patterns of relationships. The process of life will take on new meaning. As the life process in man becomes better understood, nursing is further enabled to initiate and implement positive measures directed toward achieving well-being for people.

FOOTNOTES

1. Seaborg, Glenn, "Address to the Secondary Education Board Conference," San Francisco, California, April 5, 1957.

CHAPTER 16

TRANSLATION INTO PRACTICE

"... those who have enough theoretical knowledge,
critical judgment, and discipline of learning to adapt
rapidly to the new situations and problems which constantly arise in the modern world."

—René Dubos

Nursing is both a science and an art. The science of nursing
is a body of abstract knowledge arrived at by scientific research
and logical analysis. It is this body of knowledge that encompasses nursing's descriptive, explanatory, and predictive principles
indispensable to professional practice in nursing. The practice of
nursing encompasses the art of nursing and is the utilization of
nursing's body of abstract knowledge in service to man. New
dimensions of artistry are achieved as the science of nursing grows
and is incorporated into practice.

The social ends for which nursing exists find fulfillment in
the union of theory and practice. Concomitantly, it must be kept
in mind that theory and practice are clearly different entities and
must not be confused with each other. Nor is experience a sub-
stitute for learning. Campbell has stated: "No popular saying is
more misleading than that we learn from experience; really the
capacity for learning from experience is one of the rarest gifts of
genius, attained by humble folk only by long and arduous training. . . . When we have established how little worthy of confidence
is 'practical knowledge' we shall be in a position to see the value
of theory."[1] Polanyi further emphasizes this point in the following statement: "Almost every major systematic error which has
deluded men for thousands of years relied on practical experience."[2]

A science does not emerge full blown out of a vacuum. Rather,
it progresses through prescientific stages accumulating knowledges

121

which have within them the potential for serious conceptual development. The evolution of a conceptual system and the derivation of unifying principles and hypothetical generalizations provide the basis for professional nursing practice. To understand and to cope with escalating changes in a wide range of unpredicted circumstances require broad principles and the ability to pull these together in novel ways.

Professional practice is creative and imaginative. It is rooted in abstract knowledge, intellectual judgment, and human compassion. There are no set formulas by which action is determined. Nor are there rules of thumb subject to memorization and unquestioning application. The tools of practice are numerous, but their appropriate selection according to the needs of an individual, a family, or society is dependent upon intellectual skill.

Nursing exists to serve people. Its direct and over-riding responsibility is to society. Nursing has no dependent functions but, like all other professions, it has many collaborative ones. Health services to people require the concerted action of a range of disciplines if such services are to approach safety and adequacy. But the safe practice of nursing depends on the nature and amount of scientific nursing knowledge the individual brings to practice and the imaginative, intellectual judgment with which such knowledge is made explicit in service to mankind.

Technological developments have mightily increased the range and variability of equipment pertinent to nursing practice. Indeed, so rapid are these developments that machines quickly become obsolete and practitioners must be continuously adapting to new devices. Manual skills, contributory to practice, are readily learned but their safe utilization is contingent on understanding. Nursing's conceptual frame of reference and its guiding principles provide the foundation for understanding. Human relationships as instruments of therapy are increasingly emphasized. The wholeness of man and his integrality with nature are basic premises underwriting nursing practice.

Professional practice in nursing seeks to promote symphonic interaction between man and environment, to strengthen the coherence and integrity of the human field, and to direct and redirect patterning of the human and environmental fields for realization of maximum health potential.

Maintenance and promotion of health are a nation's first line of defense in building a healthy society. Nursing's conceptual system provides a means of perceiving man and of envisioning his developmental transition. The principle of helicy specifies man's unidirectional, rhythmic complexifying and connotes direction in helping people to achieve positive health. Concomitantly, probabilistic goal setting becomes the handmaiden of the values to which man may adhere at any given point in space-time. Changing values are themselves products of helical evolution and reflect the negentropic nature of man and environment. Maintenance and promotion of health, viewed from this perspective, are more flexible, allow for greater individual differences, and are more cognizant of maturational complexities coordinate with health.

Activities of daily living must encompass opportunities for rhythmic consistency and for man-environment interchange that stimulate the flow of repatterning commensurate with the openness of nature. For example, studies of so-called sensory deprivation provide evidence of man's responses to variations in the nature and amount of specified kinds of sensory input. Overstimulation, as well as understimulation, has also been subjected to questioning. The principle of resonancy denotes a rhythmic flow of energy waves which order and reorder the human field. The man-environment relationship is a complex symmetry uniting man and environment in a universal orchestration of dynamic wave patterns. The nature, amount, and speed of wave propagation portends enhancement or disruption of man's development. Enhancement requires that there be intervention that will strengthen the man-environment symmetry.

Positive health measures will be directed toward determining individual differences and assisting people to develop patterns of living coordinate with environmental changes rather than in conflict with them. This is *not* to propose that man is simply to accept environmental changes as they occur. Rather, man and environment change together and man plays his role in directing change, both consciously and unconsciously. But, whatever goals may be set, the mutuality of the process is a significant factor in their achievement.

To maintenance and promotion of health must be added prevention and correction of health problems including those stemming from social inequities, technological advances, and other events on the public scene. Advocates of community health point to poor and inadequate housing, ghetto areas, racial and occupational discrimination, economic and educational deprivation, criminal acts, suicide rates, drug addiction, property destruction, mental retardation, and poor and inadequate delivery of health services as in critical need of public action. Legislation and funding for work with heart, cancer, and stroke conditions reflect public concern with these disorders and support a disease-oriented approach to their reduction. Mental health clinics and child guidance centers emphasize the existence of emotional disturbances. Ecological imbalances growing out of the use of pesticides, detergents, and water and air pollutants add a further dimension to man's predicament. The population explosion, artificial organ transplants, rising radiation levels, and genetic discoveries further complicate the picture.

The need for valid and substantial community health services has never been so acute. To deal with such a wide range of seemingly diverse problems as those indicated above requires the seeing of a pattern, a concept of the wholeness of man and his environment, and a recognition of escalating, dynamic evolution.

No one is exempt from the impact of environmental transition or social and health conditions. Intervention must proceed on many fronts. The principles of homeodynamics provide guidelines for the attack. A concept of man and environment continuously shaping one another, cognizance of the synchronous nature of change, and an assumption of complexifying rhythmicality foretell individual aand community health services which must possess clearly different characteristics from those presently in existence.

The human being is an integral participant in the intervention process. Nursing judgments and actions are not predicated upon disease entities, nor do they have their central focus on subsystem pathology. Categorical disease entities and subsystem pathology may constitute supplementary and relevant data which would need to be taken into account in determining a nursing diagnosis. However, such conditions do not identify either the living system or the life process. Nursing intervention is predicated upon the wholeness of man and derives its safety and effectiveness from a unified concept of human functioning. Nursing is concerned with evaluating the simultaneous states of the individual (or group) and the environment, and the preceding configurations leading up to the present. Intervention is dependent on evaluation and adds a conscious dimension to enhancing probabilistic outcomes toward a predetermined goal. The practitioner of nursing is an environmental component for the individual receiving services and is always a factor in the intervention process.

Health and illness are part of the same continuum. They are not dichotomous conditions. The multiple events taking place along life's axis denote the extent to which man is achieving his maximum health potential and vary in their expressions from greatest health to those conditions which are incompatible with maintaining life processes. The total pattern of events at any given point in space-time provides the data of nursing diagnosis. Nursing, is directed toward taking these data, evaluating them determining immediate and long-range health goals for the individual, family, and society, and initiating intervention that seems most likely to achieve these goals. The dynamic nature of life signifies continuous revision of the nature and meaning of diagnostic data and concomitant revision of interventional measures.

Nursing's conceptual model provides the frame of reference for perceiving and interpreting diagnostic data. Goal setting encompasses both preservation and enhancement of meaningful life and meaningful transition from life to death. The process of life evolves in broadly predictable ways. Guiding principles provide the basis for selecting intervention appropriate to specific goals determined on an individual basis as well as for the larger goals affecting society and the future of man. Principles provide broad generalizations by which a wide range of phenomena may be explained, future events predicted, and probabilistic outcomes of a diversity of operations anticipated. As relationships between phenomena are verified, understood, and lodged within nursing's conceptual system, predictive accuracy grows and nursing practice takes on new dimensions of safety.

Judicious and wise identification of interventive measures consonant with the diagnostic pattern and the purposes to be achieved in any given situation requires the imaginative pulling together of nursing knowledges in new ways according to the particular needs of the individual or group. Interventive measures represent implementation of the "whys" of nursing.

In the process of implementation, a variety of tools may be used to bring about and augment the efficacy of nursing practice. Thermometers, electrical monitoring devices, oxygen equipment, and a range of other mechanical contrivances of varying complexity of design and operation may be used to supplement diagnostic data and to contribute to therapeutic fruitfulness. Personal and procedural activities such as baths, exercises, injections, catheterizations, enemas, and many other such operations utilize manual and manipulative skills and constitute significant resources to be drawn upon in effecting desired changes. Intellectual skill in selecting those tools and procedures best suited to a given situation and artistry in utilization of mechanical and personal resources are important dimensions of nursing practice. However, it must be thoroughly understood that tools and procedures are adjuncts to practice and are safe and meaningful only to the extent that knowledgeable nursing judgments underwrite their selection and the ways in which they may be used.

The practical application of abstract knowledge takes many forms. What are some illustrations of the relevance of research findings for nursing practice? Felton's study (see p. 108) points out the disruption in selected indices that occurs in people experiencing a one-hour shift in social routines. An individual admitted to hospital is frequently subjected to a more drastic shift in routines than the one-hour shift investigated by Felton. Moreover, while Felton's study population maintained the same routines within the one-hour shift, the hospitalized person generally experiences changes within the routines as well as the time shift. Specifically, hospitalization, as currently experienced, may set off further disorganization of an individual's rhythmic pattern than may already exist coordinate with the reason for his hospitalization. What changes then need to be made in traditional hospital routines in order that hospitalization may enhance the integrity of the individual rather than reducing therapeutic effectiveness and possibly diminishing human safety?

Individual rhythm profiles might well become standard diagnostic data for all hospital admissions. Flexibility in hospital routines which could enable individuals to evolve reciprocal man-environment repatterning toward greater developmental coherence could be initiated. Indices other than those studied by Felton need to be identified and evaluated.

Nursing practice involves a range of behaviors, operations, and procedures. Rhythmic correlates of practice must be determined and taken into consideration in planning and implementing intervention. Such consideration has relevance for both patients and nurses. The not uncommon practice of rotating work shifts for staff nurses in hospitals suggests that such nurses may themselves be in a continuous state of arrhythmic functioning which in turn would affect their practice and might have potentially detrimental outcomes for patients. The rhythmic correlates of staffing patterns need investigation.

The motion studies reported by Neal, Porter, and Earle (see Chapter 14) support the significance of movement in infant growth and development. Although further investigations need to be done in this area, there is nonetheless support for encouraging nursing personnel and parents to provide motion opportunities for infants. Should the rocking cradle of an earlier generation be returned to the nursery? Could there be a further unexpected dividend that might accrue from exercises during pregnancy?

Fagin's study (see Chapter 14) of rooming-in for mothers of young hospitalized children is substantive evidence of the need for pediatric units in hospitals to revise policies both to make possible and to encourage mothers to stay in hospital with their children. While all mothers may not be able to remain continuously during the child's period of hospitalization, open visiting hours for mothers could be instituted and efforts made to have mothers present as much as possible. Nursing of children in hospital with mothers present would add new dimensions and enhanced opportunities for professional nurse practice in pediatric units as well as contributing to the therapeutic effectiveness of hospitalization for the child.

Nursing's conceptual model has equal relevance whether an individual is deemed to be sick or well. Behavioral manifestations are interpreted according to the principles of homeodynamics. Projected changes in the life process are determined within the context of nursing's conceptual system. The effectiveness of this approach to nursing practice is revealed in the extent to which human health and welfare are benefited.

Nursing practice focuses on human beings—on man in his entirety and wholeness. Nursing diagnosis encompasses the man-environment relationship and seeks to identify sequential, cross-sectional patterning in the life process. Nursing intervention is directed toward repatterning of man and environment for more effective fulfillment of life's capabilities. Life's capabilities encompass man's humanness, his creative promise, his capacity to feel and reason, the symphonic potential of his tangible structure and functioning.

Nursing practice must be flexible and creative, individualized and socially oriented, compassionate and skillful. Professional practitioners in nursing must be continuously translating theoretical knowledge into human service and participating in the coordination of their knowledges and skills with those of professional personnel in other health disciplines. Nursing's conceptual system provides the foundation for nursing practice. Basic and applied research in nursing furnishes the knowledges to be translated.

FOOTNOTES

1. Campbell, Norman, *What Is Science?* New York: Dover Publications, Inc., 1952, p. 170.

2. Polanyi, Michael, *Personal Knowledge,* Chicago, Illinois: The University of Chicago Press, 1958, p. 183.

CHAPTER **17**

DESIGN FOR RELEVANCE

". . . every major step forward by mankind entails some loss, the sacrifice of an older security and the creation and heightening of new tensions."

—William Barrett

Modern nursing was born of an idealism that was unafraid to face nineteenth century realities of human suffering, social irresponsibility, and inadequate and incompetent health services. In the past decade, time has kaleidoscoped with sweeping advances in science and technology. The public is demanding social and health services of a nature and quality clearly beyond that currently available—or even imagined. Automation threatens man's privacy. The immorality of human experimentation without informed consent of the individual has become a national issue—its existence so well documented that it has led to legislative action. Genetic research and artificial transplants are moving the "androids" of science fiction into the real world. Man has walked upon the moon. Roles and responsibilities of health personnel, relevant to the past, are no longer germane to the world of today and tomorrow.

On July 20, 1969 man made explicit his entry into a new era. A short sixty years after the Wright brothers gave their epoch-making exhibition of an airborne machine and less than ten years after the project for a moon landing got under way, Armstrong, Aldrin, and Collins gave reality to man's age-old dream of travel to other worlds.

Man is no longer bound to planet Earth. Older cosmologies do not suffice to explain the nature of man and his becoming. Basic assumptions underlying contemporary health services are disintegrating in the face of new knowledges and new interpretations

129

of man and his environment. Society cannot afford the narrow, un-imaginative, and inadequately conceived expansion of sick services, no matter how well intentioned, except as these become subsidiary to the larger purposes of maintaining and promoting human health and welfare. Nor can continuation of the traditional focus on cate-gorical diseases contribute meaningfully to man's well-being. Dis-ease entities must be subsumed within the larger perspective of ecological relationships. The complementarity of man and environ-ment must become explicit throughout the gamut of health and welfare services, whether directed toward habilitation or reha-bilitation.

An increasingly better informed public is demanding partici-pation in determining the nature and quality of public services—in education, in health, in welfare, in government, and in other areas of human life. And though the public expects that each profes-sional discipline possesses scientific knowledge of potential public benefit, they are distrustful (and with some reason) of authoritarian control by vested interests wherever these may be found. The nature and delivery of health services are under serious scrutiny. Questionable practices, excessive charges, and a critical shortage of trained personnel are receiving national attention. A range of pro-grams have been designed, hopefully to alleviate these problems, but too often such programs have been poorly conceived or badly implemented.

Professionally educated nurses carry a real responsibility for exercising significant leadership in envisioning, initiating, and im-plementing health services commensurate with present knowledge and directed toward an unknown future. For example, though crit-ically needed, current activity toward making community-based diagnostic and treatment centers readily accessible to people is primarily limited to providing medical care, and makes little or no provision for comprehensive health services which require the inclusion of personnel from a range of fields other than medicine (i.e., professional nursing, clinical psychology, social work, dentistry, and others, one of which I would suggest should be podiatry). Furthermore, there is critical need to incorporate within commun-ity-based centers services designed to maintain and promote health (not to be confused with prevention of disease) and to transmute the present limited ventures into truly community health resources.

For more than a century nurses have provided community-based (home, school, etc.) health services through a range of public

health agencies—voluntary and tax supported, rural and urban—
for people who were well and for those who were sick. The scope
of professional education in nursing has traditionally encompassed
man wherever he might be and whatever his state of health. Major
advances in public health measures have come about through nursing leaders whose social concern and foresight were pre-eminent,
from Florence Nightingale to the present.

Organized "home care" services have existed for many decades.
It is therefore strange that, in recent years, proposals to initiate
such services with no apparent awareness of their long existence
have emerged and are duplicating already existing services. The
nature and delivery of health services would be better served by
the imaginative development of means for expanding, enhancing,
and revising existing services than by engaging in uninformed and
wasteful duplication of present services.

The critical shortage of nursing personnel is primarily a shortage of professionally educated nurses and an obsolete system that
results in misuse of both professional and technical registered nurses.
An unwitting public is being victimized by the addition of massive
numbers of unskilled and minimally skilled persons to give nursing
care at the same time that registered nurses are forced by the "system" to spend one-half of their time in non-nursing activities. Many
of these non-nursing duties are properly the responsibility of other
kinds of personnel and other areas of a hospital. Installation of
automated equipment could substantially reduce non-nursing activities, increase registered nurse hours to patients, and enhance both
technical and professional nursing practice. Professionally educated
practitioners are not only spending much time in non-nursing
operations but, unless they are watchful, they find themselves denied
opportunity to practice at the level of their preparation and to
provide the knowledgeable judgments indispensable to public safety
and beyond the ken of nursing's technical practitioners (graduates
of associate degree and hospital school programs). Professional and
technical registered nurses are no more interchangeable than are
dentists and dental hygienists or medical doctors and medical tech-
nicians.

Multiple examples can be found of contemporary difficulties
with which a design for relevance must grapple. Critical problems
of everyday life have roused a world population to demand that
human beings shall be better fed, housed, and clothed; that all
people shall enjoy the fruits of science and technology; and that

opportunities for education and health shall be equally available to everyone. The process of achieving such utopian goals, however, suffers from too frequent efforts to use nineteenth century solutions for twentieth century problems when even twentieth century solutions are notably inadequate. Counts's comment that "as our feet tread the earth of a new world our heads continue to dwell in the past"[1] is sadly pertinent to the contemporary scene, despite a manned moon landing. Equally shortsighted are those who propose that man must first solve the problems of this planet *before* continuing his exploration of space.

A perception of man's planet-bound past must give way to a realization of his space-directed future. Such a view is by no means a denial of critical need to promote well-being for man in his planetary existence on Earth. It *is* a proposal that the unfolding of existence on Earth is integrally bound with man's advent into a new dimension of the universe. Recognition of ecological relationships must be extended to encompass ecological changes already set in motion by man's yet primitive space travel. The reality of man's negentropic complexifying is a promise of unfulfilled potentialities.

A design for relevance must be rooted in a philosophy of the creativity of life and a belief in man's evolutionary future. Change is inevitable. A constructive approach to achieving human health and welfare must replace the generally fear-inducing taboos that emphasize avoidance of practices speculated to reduce longevity. Health services of the future need to incorporate emphasis on practices that can enhance life.

Nursing's conceptual system adds a critically needed dimension to the broad field of health and welfare. With the formulation of nursing principles, the way is opened to a range of investigations of conditions under which particular principles hold. As the validity and reliability of these principles are verified, their value in guiding nursing practice becomes more explicit. The translation of scientific nursing knowledge into humanitarian practice carries with it the potential for health services of markedly enlarged scope and greater public safety than are currently available.

Professional personnel concerned with public health and welfare must develop mutual respect for the knowledge and skills possessed by the various health fields and recognition that, today, even safe health services require the concerted efforts of several disciplines for their provision. No one discipline holds the key to human health and welfare nor is any one discipline competent to determine the purposes and actions of any other discipline. In the process of equal sharing between professional fields, the potential emerges for transcending the capabilities of any one of these fields and of evolving socially oriented goals relevant to the future of mankind.

The citizenry must be directly involved in development and implementation of services affecting their well-being. Individual rights to informed consent of persons subjected to experimental procedures are only partially protected by law. Governmental provisions for more widespread availability of services to the sick are being jeopardized by unexplained discrepancies between charges and costs. Respect for human dignity and individual differences, of paramount importance if today's problems are to be dealt with effectively, is in grave need of augmentation. Many of those who cry for law and order ignore social injustices that underlie upheaval. Mental health clinics multiply at the same time that factors contributory to emotional problems continue.

That the evolution of man might be undergoing significant acceleration concurrent with escalating advances in science and technology has received little attention. Concomitantly, the unidirectional, synchronous complexifying of man and environment postulated in this volume finds expression in innovative repatterning of both. In general, environmental events tend to be evaluated according to whether they seem to be immediately harmful or not harmful to human life. Long-range and evolutionary implications of these events are commonly ignored.

Health services must be designed to take into account evolutionary escalation in both man and environment. Ecological relationships are undergoing major revisions with many unanticipated consequences. Patterns of health and illness reveal numerous changes in recent decades. Social turmoil exists world wide. Youth is demanding major educational reforms. More persons are surviving to old age.

Man is readying himself for life in a new dimension—that of outer space and other worlds. Space hospitals are nearing the launching pad. As well as caring for space travelers, such hospitals may well provide a therapeutic environment for persons having cardiac problems, emotional disturbances, and other conditions. Ability to provide varying levels of gravity will add further dimensions to the armamentarium of intervention. Future generations may not need the extensive life support systems used by today's astronauts. (Or it might be proposed that there will be those who might need life support systems in reverse.)

Health problems cannot be separated from the world's social ills. Neither can they be dealt with effectively by means of disease-oriented measures. Fear campaigns, though extensive, accomplish little in changing habits proposed to be harmful to health. Short-sighted interpretations of statistical correlations in the absence of a philosophy of the nature of life and its becoming set in motion short-lived and dubious recommendations for health practices. Health fads vie with professional advice and achieve a large public following. Criticisms of critical inadequacy in the delivery of health services are rampant, but even more serious should be concern with the nature of that which is delivered.

The resolution of health problems and the setting of goals directed toward achieving a healthy people require a new concept of the unity of man and a recognition of man's capacity to feel and to reason. Man possesses major resources within himself for determining direction in the developmental process. People must be informed and active participants in the search for health. Intervention should be directed toward assisting individuals to mobilize their resources, consciously and unconsciously, so that the man-environment relationship may be strengthened and the integrity of the individual heightened. Therapeutic modalities must incorporate within them cognizance of man as a thinking, feeling being. Humanitarian goals are needed to motivate health services.

A design for relevance requires the seeing of a pattern. Nursing's conceptual system provides a frame of reference for evolving a new approach to the nature and delivery of health services. Vision and imagination must attend the development of health resources and the determination of both short- and long-range goals coordinate with present and anticipated knowledge. The education of nursing's professional practitioners must emphasize general education and broad principles that can be translated into human service in novel and unpredicted ways. Graduate education in nursing must be revised to incorporate a basic focus on the life process in man with specialty areas evolving out of man's developmental wholeness. Scholars and scientists in nursing must pursue the exciting task of evolving new knowledge and of incorporating it into the instructional process in order that it may find its way into socially significant action.

With the emergence of a body of scientific knowledge in nursing, new potentials for meaningful service to mankind reconfirm nursing's long commitment to human health and welfare. A common purpose, that of helping people achieve maximum well-being within the capability of each person, constitutes a strong unifying force for all who nurse. Commitment to nursing as a social necessity binds nurses together. Concern for human beings draws new recruits into nursing. Opportunity to act out that concern in human service, according to one's knowledge and preparation, keeps people in nursing. Knowledgeable nursing services have a socially significant contribution to make to man's future, whatever that future may hold.

FOOTNOTES

1. Counts, George S., "The Impact of Technological Change," *The Planning of Change*, New York: Holt, Rinehart and Winston, 1962, p. 21.

RELATED READINGS

ANDREWS, DONALD H., *The Symphony of Life*, Lee's Summit, Mo.: Unity Books, 1966.

ARENDT, HANNAH, *The Human Condition*, Garden City, N. Y.: Doubleday & Co., Inc., 1958.

ASIMOV, ISAAC, *Understanding Physics: Motion, Sound, and Heat*, London: George Allen & Unwin, Ltd., 1966.

———, *Understanding Physics: Light, Magnetism, and Electricity*, London: George Allen & Unwin, Ltd., 1966.

———, *Understanding Physics: The Electron, Proton, and Neutron*, London: George Allen & Unwin, Ltd., 1966.

Bergman, Peter G., *The Riddle of Gravitation*, New York: Charles Scribner's Sons, 1968.

BERRIEN, F. KENNETH, *General and Social Systems*, New Brunswick, N. J.: Rutgers University Press, 1968.

BERTHOLD, JEANNE S., "Theoretical and Empirical Clarification of Concepts," *Nursing Science*, Vol. 2, No. 5, October 1964, pp. 406-422.

BUNGE, MARIO, *Intuition and Science*, Englewood Cliffs, N. J.: Prentice-Hall, Inc., 1962.

CHESTER, MICHAEL, *Relativity: An Introduction for Young Readers*, New York: W. W. Norton & Co., Inc., 1967.

CROWTHER, J. G., *The Sciences of Energy*, London: Frederick Muller, Ltd., 1954.

DANTO, A. and MORGENBESSER, S. (Edit.), *Philosophy of Science*, New York: Meridian Books, Inc., 1960.

DUBOS, RENÉ, *The Dreams of Reason,* New York: Columbia University Press, 1961.

————, *So Human an Animal,* New York: Charles Scribner's Sons, 1968.

DUNN, HALBERT, "Man, Energy, and the Life Process," *MAIN CURRENTS in Modern Thought,* Vol. 15, No. 1, September 1958.

FISCHER, ROLAND (Edit.), *Interdisciplinary Perspectives of Time,* New York: New York Academy of Science, 1967.

GATES, DAVID, *Energy Exchange in the Biosphere,* New York: Harper and Row, 1962

GLASER, B and STRAUSS, A., *The Discovery of Grounded Theory: Strategies for Qualitative Research,* Chicago: Aldine Publishing Company, 1967.

HEMPEL, CARL G., *Fundamentals of Concept Formation in Empirical Science,* Chicago: University of Chicago Press, 1952.

KERLINGER, FRED, *Foundations of Behavioral Research,* New York: Holt, Rinehart and Winston, Inc., 1964.

KRIEGER, DOLORES, "About the Life Process," *Nursing Science,* Vol. 1, No. 2, June 1963, pp. 105-115.

LEHNINGER, ALBERT L., *Bioenergetics,* New York: W. A. Benjamin, Inc., 1965.

LERNER, DANIEL (Edit.), *Evidence and Inference,* Glencoe, Ill.: The Free Press, 1962.

MASLOW, ABRAHAM H., *The Psychology of Science,* New York: Harper and Row, 1966.

PLATT, JOHN R. (Edit.), *New Views of the Nature of Man,* Chicago: The University of Chicago Press, 1965.

POLANYI, MICHAEL, *Personal Knowledge.* Chicago: The University of Chicago Press, 1958.

POPPER, KARL, *The Logic of Scientific Discovery,* New York: Harper and Row, 1965.

PUTNAM, PHYLLIS, "A Conceptual Approach to Nursing Theory," *Nursing Science,* Vol. 3, No. 6, December 1965, pp. 430-442.

ROGERS, MARTHA E., *Reveille in Nursing,* Philadelphia: F. A. Davis Company, 1964.

STEBBING, L. SUSAN, *A Modern Elementary Logic,* New York: Barnes & Noble, 1961.

TARSKI, ALFRED, *Introduction to Logic,* New York: Oxford University Press, 1946.

EPILOGUE

"What is past is prologue."

—National Archives Building
Washington, D.C.

A Washington tourist passing the National Archives Building is reported to have asked her cab driver the meaning of the inscription; "What is past is prologue." His response, "Lady, it means you ain't seen nothin' yet", is a remarkably simple prophecy of wonders still to take place.

Nursing's scientific coming of age is an expression of changing times and new approaches to cosmic understanding. The story of life's emergence out of the dim recesses of the past gives credence to man's evolutionary future. Accelerating change in both man and environment bespeaks a new threshold in man's transition as he readies himself for extraterrestrial living. Grim predictions of potential dangers to be found in manned flights to other worlds become less dire as healthy astronauts report greater ease of locomotion on the moon than on Earth. Heavy emphasis has been placed on the perils of bringing harmful organisms to this planet, but little has been noted of the ecological benefits and innovative potentials to be derived from man's entry into outer space.

Many troubles beset the peoples of Earth and cry for resolution. Social and economic inequities abound. Multiple deviations from health affect many persons. The "population explosion" and increasing numbers of individuals who are living their full three score years and ten portend a rapidly diminishing per capita of available space. Ethical decisions of far-reaching import are in the making as genetic research, artificial organ transplants, human experimentation, and governmental depersonalization grow.

Technological successes make possible rapid and world-wide communication. Large numbers of people are bypassing centuries of Western World development as modern transportation carries men and knowledge to all parts of the globe. Despite vying ideologies and widespread nationalism, the peoples of the world are drawn together as never before.

Atmospheric changes proceed apace in the wake of vehicular exhaust fumes (ground and air), radiation fallout, industrial smog, chemical sprays, man-made electrical discharges, volcanic gases, and a wide range of other largely unrecognized phenomena. Primitive man's atmospheric envelope was very different from that surroundin modern man. Today's environmental complexities incorporate within them ever more rapid alteration in the composition of the air man breathes.

Everyday life encompasses extraordinary speeds scarcely dreamed of half a century ago. Population concentrations attend urbanization and an international diet is replacing local food habits. In many areas production rises as man-hours of work decrease. Major inadequacies and irrelevancies in education and training come into view as employment opportunities undergo radical shifts and swift revisions. Tomorrow's employables must possess broad knowledge, flexibility, and the capacity to use learning in novel ways.

The creativity of life finds expression in man's expanding awareness of the universe and a growing capacity to know his world through paranormal means. Thought and feelings portray man's humanness and underwrite his search for meaning. A wakenning humanitarianism grows despite special interests and promulgators of dissidence. The world's problems in health, education, and welfare must be seen within the context of the incredible magnificence of man's potentials.

The moving boundaries of nursing have advanced through a prescientific era to a dawning, scientifically based humanitarianism that holds within it the promise of new and expanded benefits to mankind. Nursing is a learned profession. Professional education is characterized by the transmission of a body of abstract principles arrived at by scientific research and logical analysis. An organized conceptual system provides the frame of reference from which testable hypotheses can evolve and in which the findings of research can be lodged. Nursing's body of scientific knowledge is specific to nursing and encompasses nursing's descriptive, explanatory, and predictive principles indispensable to professional practice. The essentiality of nursing's abstract system is not a proposal that technical skills are unimportant. Rather, technical skills are tools which, when used with intellectual judgment and applied with artistry, augment the translation of theory into socially significant service to human beings.

The principles of homeodynamics encompass a way of perceiving man and his world and provide guidlines for predicting the nature and direction of man's development. Health and illness are merged within man's synergistic wholeness. Deviations along life's axis issue out of the synchronous complementarity of man and environment. Interventive measures seek to strengthen the integrity of the man-environment relationship and to give direction to man's struggle to achieve new levels of well-being.

The science of nursing must be made explicit in research, education, and practice. Interdisciplinary sharing, directed toward developing imaginative and forward-looking designs that can lead to improving human health and welfare, must engage professional personnel in all of the health fields. Responsible leadership must emerge and take on the great task of evolving health services commensurate with a world in rapid transition and committed to humanitarian goals. There is no going back. New horizons call. Nursing has moved into a new era of fulfilling human needs.

INDEX